Hormone Replacement Therapy

Hormone Replacement Therapy

Your Guide to Making an Informed Choice

Rosemary Nicol

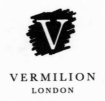

VERMILION
LONDON

Published in 1993 by Vermilion
an imprint of Ebury Press
Random House
20 Vauxhall Bridge Road
London SW1V 2SA

Catalogue record for this book is available
from the British Library.

ISBN 0 09 177666 X

Typeset in Baskerville by Hope Services (Abingdon) Ltd.
Printed and bound in Great Britain by
Mackays of Chatham Plc, Kent

The contents of this book are for information only and are
intended to assist readers in identifying medical symptoms and
conditions. The book is not intended to be a substitute for taking
proper medical advice and should not be relied upon in this
way. *Always* consult a duly qualified doctor. The author and
publisher cannot accept responsibility for illness arising out of
the failure to seek medical advice from a doctor.

To David, with love

Contents

Chapter 1

'It's just your age . . .'

‘Nowadays, we think we know all there is to know about sex, having babies, contraception, and all that. Yet we seem to know so little about the menopause. I thought it was just a few hot flushes and no more periods. Why don't we talk about it more, compare notes, learn from each other? We do about most other things.’

Talking about the menopause is something that most women have just never done. We talk about other aspects of our lives, but not this one. As a result, a conspiracy of shame and silence has drifted down the generations, expressed in such phrases as: 'It's her time of life', 'She's going through the Change, poor old thing', 'Take no notice of her, she's just having a hot flush'. Say no more, nudge nudge, wink wink.

Now, however, at last, compared with their predecessors, women reaching the menopause could be the lucky ones, the ones who know about it and are well informed. They can recognise hot flushes and other symptoms for what they are: the body's response to a fall in the level of the female hormone oestrogen – simply that. They are not something shameful; nor do they mean we are suddenly old. After all, who wants to feel old at 50? It will be another 30 years before you need even to start worrying about that, so don't wish it on yourself now.

Part of the problem is that, until fairly recently, the majority of women didn't live long enough to experience the menopause. Until reliable birth control became readily available, women who bore children tended to spend the majority of their married lives in a state of pregnancy or breast-feeding until their early forties. A combination of continuing pregnancies and the hazards of childbirth, as well as poor sanitation and inadequate health care, meant that, even at the start of the twentieth century, most women were dead by about fifty. So it is hardly surprising that so little was known about the menopause, let alone talked about.

Those who did survive to the menopause never made much of a fuss about it. They used a bit of self-medication, herbal remedies handed down through the generations, or exciting dietary supplements like 'two sheep's ovaries a day sandwiched between unleavened bread', or 'one tankard daily of the urine of a she-goat', and waited for it to pass.

Today, we often feel the menopause is just another illness to be treated by visits to the doctor and by medication. We hear the term 'deficiency disease', that is we are deficient in oestrogen. Yet most women still don't really know what the menopause is, when it might happen, what to expect, and what can be done to ease their passage through it.

The Menopause

Small children notice fairly quickly that girls are not like boys, and women are not like men. They are different shapes, have different bits, later on they have different types of voices and hair in different places. During the late teens and early twenties, the superficial differences may become blurred – one person with a pony tail and earrings may be male, another with cropped hair and jeans may be female – but as long as they themselves know which is which, who are we to criticise?

From the moment of conception, the foetus is programmed to develop the type of hormones that will give him or her male or female characteristics. A hormone is a substance produced by glands in one part of the body, which causes changes to occur in other parts of the body. The male child produces more of the male hormone, testosterone, and the female child more of the female hormones, the oestrogens (pronounced 'eestrojens'). In fact, we all produce some quantities of both male and female hormones, but from puberty onwards 'our own' particular hormone starts to predominate and we develop the outward visible signs of one gender or the other.

At puberty, a boy's level of testosterone starts to rise. As a result, his voice gets deeper, he develops facial hair, and his bones and muscles become bigger and stronger. At puberty, a girl's level of oestrogen (in a form called oestradiol) starts to rise and, among other things, her periods start, her breasts develop and her body takes on a rounder shape. During the years of menstruation we tend to regard the monthly bleed as the only sign of hormonal changes occurring, but the levels of our various hormones go up and down throughout the menstrual cycle, and what we know as the menstrual period is the body's visible response to these many changes.

The female hormones

Oestrogen is produced in the ovaries, and causes changes to occur in the breasts, uterus (womb), cervix, vagina, skin and hair, blood, bones, and even the mind. It affects so many parts of a woman's body that it is not surprising that we really notice the changes that occur when the level starts to fall at the time of the menopause.

All of the essentially 'female' organs contain oestrogen receptors, which respond to the presence of oestrogen in the body. This means that, while oestrogen levels are normal, the breasts are firm and full; the walls of the vagina are thick and elastic, and able to secret mucus (especially during sexual intercourse); skin texture is firm; and bones are strong. Oestrogen also keeps blood vessels healthy, produces a feeling of wellbeing, and contributes to sex-drive. During those periods of a woman's life when her oestrogen levels

are high (especially during the middle months of pregnancy), she will look and feel absolutely terrific. 'Glowing'
and 'radiant' are words typically used, reflecting the fact
that a woman's hair is lustrous, her skin blooms, and she
radiates a feeling of wellbeing and contentment. After the
baby is born, some women's oestrogen levels fall so low that
their hair and skin suffer badly, and the feeling of wellbeing
may be replaced by postnatal depression.

The other important hormone of the female reproductive
cycle is progesterone; it is produced each month by the
ovaries after ovulation (the production of an egg) has taken
place. The main functions of progesterone are to prepare
the womb for a fertilised egg (ovum) and to maintain pregnancy. Progesterone works with the oestrogens to cause the
lining of the womb to thicken in preparation for a fertilised
egg. If fertilisation does not occur, the lining of the womb
comes away in the form of the monthly period.

How the menopause begins

As the menopause approaches, eggs are produced by the
ovaries less regularly, leading to irregular levels of oestrogen
and then to an overall decline in the average amount of
oestrogen produced each month. (The number of ovarian
follicles, and the egg cells they contain, decreases steadily
from birth onwards, accelerating after about the age of 35,
until by the time of the menopause, only a few egg cells
remain.) As ovulation becomes less frequent, the ovaries
produce no more progesterone, the lining of the womb no
longer thickens each month and periods cease.

Eventually, the time comes when the ovaries produce
almost no oestrogen or progesterone, although they continue to produce hormones called androgens. Androgens (of
which testosterone is an example) are hormones that produce male characteristics, but these androgens definitely
belong in the female body, and influence general health,
sexuality and muscular strength. Some androgens are con-
verted to oestrogen in the body's fat cells, so women with

more fat produce more oestrogen after the menopause and may have fewer problems with hot flushes, vaginal dryness and osteoporosis than thinner women. So there is some advantage in having that extra body fat! The disadvantage is that overweight women may produce too much oestrogen, and run an increased risk of developing cancer of the womb or breast. Although all women will be producing some oestrogen from the adrenal glands, there is not enough after the menopause to keep bones strong, prevent menopausal symptoms and protect against arterial disease.

Until the menopause, a woman's natural level of oestrogens is very much higher than her natural level of androgens. Once the menopause has passed, oestrogens fall to a very low level but androgens continue to be produced; this may explain why older women sometimes develop increased facial hair and their voices deepen slightly.

The coming of the menopause doesn't mean you are now 'unfemale', or unfeminine, or old, unless *you* let it affect you that way. If you tell people you feel less female, they will start to view you that way; if you start to look, behave and dress like an old woman, people will treat you as old. There are so many advantages to reaching the time of the menopause, it would be a pity to let society's view of older women spoil it all. You have now left behind you the difficulties of looking after young children, you are almost certainly more confident and self-assured than you were 20 years ago; your periods have ended, and with them premenstrual tension, pelvic aching, cramps, tampons, and the need for using birth control. You are probably better off financially than when you had children and a building society to support, and as family responsibilities lessen there is more time for new interests and activities. The end of fertility does not mean the end of your attractiveness as a person; it can mean a whole new era of your life dawning, full of possibilities for fulfilment that were unattainable when you were younger. In the days when most women didn't live that long, the menopause meant old age; now women have at least another 30 years left to live, years full of new opportunities.

When does the menopause happen?

❝I heard that the earlier you start your periods the earlier they finish.❞

❝Oh, I thought it was just the opposite, that the earlier you started the later you finish.❞

When used by doctors, the term 'menopause' means, literally, 'last menstrual period', but women use it to mean that whole period of their lives between first starting to experience menopausal symptoms, such as hot flushes, and the end of their periods and the troublesome symptoms. Doctors use the word 'climacteric' to describe this period (from the Greek *klimakter*, meaning 'a critical period'), and they divide it loosely into three phases:

Pre-menopause When periods are still regular, but the first symptoms may appear – usually hot flushes and mood changes.

Peri-menopause When the ovaries' function declines, periods become irregular, and symptoms either start or become troublesome. This leads up to the time of the last menstrual period.

Post-menopause From the time of a woman's last period until the end of her days.

The problem with the concept of a 'last menstrual period' is that a woman doesn't know she has had her last period until quite a long time afterwards. Was that last period the last one, or will you get another one in several months' time? It's not until about a year has passed without a period that it is safe to say you have finished. Consequently, the period of time we call the menopause (and doctors call the climacteric) has no clear beginning or end. For some women it will last only a year, for most about two to three years, but about one quarter of all women will still be experiencing 'short-term' menopausal symptoms five or more years after they began.

It isn't known exactly what determines the age at which a woman reaches the menopause. Nutrition is important; poor nutrition brings it on earlier. Women who have never borne children tend to have an earlier menopause than women who have had several children, and those whose last pregnancy occurred before their late twenties reputedly have an earlier menopause than those whose last pregnancy was in their thirties. Smokers reach the menopause up to five years earlier than non-smokers, probably because smoking lowers oestrogen levels, and 'passive smokers' (non-smokers who live or work amongst smokers) also tend to have an earlier menopause.

As a rough guide, most women (though by no means all) will experience the menopause at about the same time as their mothers or older female relatives did. But how do you know when that was? It's highly likely that neither your mother nor your elderly aunts ever discussed with you their experiences of the menopause; hopefully, you will feel better able to talk to your daughter about it than your mother did to you.

It is safe to say, however, that at some time in your middle years, things will start to change. It is most likely to happen around the mid to late forties, occasionally in the early fifties, and in some women it can happen as early as their thirties. Although the age at which girls start their periods has got earlier over the last few hundred years, the average age for the menopause still remains at about 50. In the third century BC, Aristotle noticed that women couldn't have children after about the age of 50. In the Middle Ages, the age was put at 50-ish, and it is still that today. We can still expect to end our reproductive days at about the same age our pre-Christian forebears did, despite the fact that our expectation of life has more than doubled since then.

The first thing a woman is most likely to notice is her periods becoming more irregular. The time between them may be less than usual or they may be further apart; they may last for a longer or shorter time; be heavier or lighter; or a combination of all these, varying from month to month. Very occasionally, a woman says she had a period at the expected time and then never had another, but this is unusual; irregular and unpredictable is how things are likely to be for quite a while.

(A small warning here: It's quite normal to have irregular periods at regular intervals, or normal periods at irregular intervals, but continual 'spotting' between periods is something to see your doctor about.)

The next stage is to miss one or more, even several, periods completely. The menstrual loss may be less than normal, even scanty, but as long as periods continue, ovulation is still taking place and pregnancy is still possible. Gradually, the gap between periods increases and the duration of bleeding becomes less and less, until a woman might think, 'Hurray, it's all over.' She may be right – or she may suddenly get another period months and months later (often at a most awkward time, such as during a holiday on a remote Greek island with the nearest chemist's shop a three-hour boat trip away!). The moral is: If you are under 50 and have had no periods for *two years*, or over 50 and have had none for *one year*, then you can probably relax; otherwise, never go away without being prepared! (This rule of thumb also applies to the likelihood of becoming pregnant, but is probably unnecessarily cautious.)

The timescale over which all these changes occur varies greatly from one woman to another, so this is one instance where your friends' experiences may not be very helpful. It is highly likely that during this time you will be experiencing a whole range of menopausal symptoms that you might feel unprepared for. The more you know about them – and what can be done about them – the more confident you will feel in yourself, and your self-confidence and self-esteem are less likely to suffer. Research has shown that many of those who find it hard to cope at this time just don't realise what's happening to them, or why, or what can be done to help them. The women who cope best are those who understand about the menopause and are able to develop a positive attitude to managing it.

Many women say, 'I've had a hysterectomy. How will this affect my menopause?' The answer is that it depends on the sort of hysterectomy you had. It is surprising how many women have no idea how much of their body was removed during their hysterectomy. Was it just the uterus (womb), or the uterus and cervix, or all that and the ovaries as well? To anyone reading this book who may have a hysterectomy at some time in the future (and to those who are still in touch with the hospital who carried out their hysterectomy in the past), it is advisable to *know your body*. In other words, don't just let 'them' do things to you unless you know what it is, and why. Surgeons who would be very reluctant to remove a man's testicles (where the male hormones are produced) will whip out a woman's ovaries (where the female hormones are produced) in the twinkling of an eye, and she may never know. So *ask*, because it will greatly affect the next few months and years of your life.

There are two sorts of menopause: a natural menopause and a surgical menopause. With a natural menopause, hormone levels gradually fall over quite a long timespan and symptoms build up slowly. This usually happens between the mid-forties and mid-fifties, though it can start much earlier and end rather later. A surgical menopause is not gradual. You may have been on the waiting list for a hysterectomy for weeks (or even months), but as far as your body is concerned it is a sudden event. One minute you have all those female bits inside you, and an hour or so later they have gone.

If you still have your ovaries, you will continue to produce oestrogen. Without a uterus, however, you will have no periods, so you won't be aware of the irregular and unpredictable winding down of periods that heralds the natural menopause. Eventually, your ovaries will start to produce less oestrogen, and you will begin to notice the typical menopausal signs, such as hot flushes. This will probably happen up to two years earlier than it might have done if you hadn't had a hysterectomy because it is thought that the uterus may release certain hormones which control levels of oestrogen, and without a uterus these oestrogen-controlling hormones are no longer produced. Many quite young women stop producing oestrogen within two or three years of a hysterectomy, even though they still have their ovaries.

If you had just one ovary removed (a unilateral oophorectomy) you may continue to produce some oestrogen. **If you had both ovaries removed** (a bi-lateral oophorectomy) you will no longer produce any oestrogen; this operation produces an instant menopause. For this reason, ask the surgeon who performs your hysterectomy to discuss with you beforehand whether he will remove the ovaries, and if so, why. Many surgeons remove them at the time of the hysterectomy to ensure that they won't become cancerous in later years. This is a valid medical point, but to remove otherwise healthy functioning ovaries can cause severe menopausal symptoms after the operation. If you have this operation before the normal menopausal age, the loss of oestrogen can produce a striking and rapid appearance of menopausal symptoms. These symptoms are so severe that it is almost certain that you will be prescribed hormone replacement therapy (HRT) straight away. If you are not, ask for it, and be prepared to keep taking it until about five years or more past what would have been your normal menopausal age, that is until you are about 55, or longer if you get on well with it. The sudden fall in oestrogen also increases the risk of developing the serious bone disease osteoporosis (see Chapter 6).

A premature menopause – whether natural or surgical – is one which occurs before about the age of 45; some doctors say before 40. If you have a premature menopause you have a greatly increased risk of developing osteoporosis and also arterial diseases that could lead to heart attacks and strokes, and you should seriously consider taking HRT from the time your premature menopause or hysterectomy or oophorectomy occurs, and be prepared to take it until you are about 55. The National Osteoporosis Society (see page 126) reports that of women aged 60–65 who have osteoporosis, a disproportionately high number had a premature menopause.

Chapter 2

Hot flushes and all that – the signs of the menopause

It is normal and natural to lose oestrogen at the time of the menopause. If, like our forebears, we didn't live much beyond the age of 50-ish, this wouldn't cause many problems. Just as women in past ages were starting to get hot flushes and night sweats, along would come the Grim Reaper and their troubles in this world would be over. Few would live to experience the long-term effects of low oestrogen, such as osteoporosis, heart attacks and strokes.

We have looked at how and why oestrogen and progesterone levels fall. Now we will look at what effect this has, and why replacing these hormones – in the form of hormone replacement therapy (HRT) – can help.

Most women probably know about hot flushes, unpredictable moods and loss of sex drive, but what else might there be?

‘You won't believe this, but I just didn't realise my problems were due to the menopause. Of course I recognised the hot flushes, but not anything else. Over the course of 18 months I lost count of the number of times I went to my doctor – we got sick of the sight of each other. I went to him about pains in my joints (he gave me paracetamol), about insomnia and night sweats (he suggested a milky bedtime drink and sleeping tablets), depression ('Why not do some charity work?'). Each time he just sighed and reached for his prescription pad, and I went away feeling a complete hypochondriac. There were other things I decided not to see him about, such as sexual difficulties and general mood changes. I couldn't understand what was happening to me as I'd been such a normal, healthy person. Luckily one day I saw another doctor in the practice. She explained that all these things were probably due to the menopause, and she talked to me about HRT, gave me a check-up (which proved I was quite normal!), and I've been on HRT ever since. **9**

The consequences of low or falling oestrogen are grouped in three categories: (a) early symptoms that, for most women, last between about six months and two years, (b) rather later symptoms that tend to become more noticeable as the years go by, and (c) conditions that may not start for many years and then get steadily worse.

Early symptoms of the menopause

These symptoms occur during the early months (or years) of the menopause when periods are erratic and unpredictable, but haven't yet stopped. Typical symptoms at this time are:

- hot flushes
- night sweats
- anxiety
- irritability
- loss of self-esteem
- difficulty in making decisions
- loss of interest in sex
- formication (see page 23)

- insomnia
- mood changes
- forgetfulness
- poor memory
- loss of confidence
- feelings of unworthiness
- headaches
- genital itching

Most of these symptoms will last for a comparatively short time, but they *can* go on for many years and can greatly reduce a woman's quality of life.

Hot flushes and night sweats

6I think I must be one of the lucky ones. When my periods first became erratic I often felt extraordinarily warm in my body and face, and sometimes I woke in the night and pushed the bedclothes off. This continued until about my last period, then never happened again. I can truthfully say I was never really bothered by hot flushes. **9**

6As a secondary school teacher, my hot flushes were so embarrassing that I nearly resigned. You can't imagine what it is like to be standing in front of a class of 15-year-olds, and suddenly to feel yourself become bright red in the face, and then to feel the sweat just running down your face. You wouldn't believe the unkind remarks they made, and more than once I ran out the classroom in tears. Within a couple of months of taking HRT the flushes had stopped, and I was back to my old self again. **9**

6I remember standing in a supermarket checkout queue. Gradually this feeling of heat spread up from my chest to my face; I know I must have gone red because the girl on the till said, "Are you alright?" It doesn't sound much to complain about, but I felt so embarrassed. Then it happened again when I was in the shops, and then again. In the end I was so afraid that I would get one of the hot flushes when I was out that I just stayed in, and my children did the shopping for me. After that I hardly left the house for three years. **9**

Hot flushes and night sweats belong in a category of symptoms that doctors call 'vasomotor symptoms', that is they are concerned with the blood vessels dilating and constricting, and with the flow of blood through these vessels. The symptoms are harmless, but most women greatly dislike having them, and find them uncomfortable, embarrassing and unpleasant. They may also affect a woman's ability to cope at work and at home, and she may even avoid social contact for fear of feeling ashamed.

The typical hot flush starts as an unpleasant sensation of heat in the face, neck or body. If it starts in the face or neck, it will probably spread down to the main part of the body; if it starts there it will spread up to the face. Often the face becomes red, and sweat appears; but many women find, to their surprise, that, despite the feelings of great heat in their face, there are no outward signs at all, and nobody has noticed.

Flushes may occur at intervals from several each hour, to just a few times each month, usually in the days leading up to the start of a period. There will be times when flushes occur frequently, and times when they do not occur at all. Each flush may last for a few seconds, or for up to half an hour, or more, but most last for about three minutes. After a flush, you may feel sweaty, then cold, and you may seem to be endlessly taking clothes off and putting them on again to get comfortable. Flushes can occur at any time of the day or night, and may be accompanied by heart palpitations, dizziness and feelings of faintness. In America, they are called 'hot flashes', but this is a less appropriate name, as it suggests something that comes and goes very rapidly. The British term 'hot flush' describes more accurately the feeling of heat that builds up and dies down slowly.

When flushes occur at night, they are called 'night sweats'. Typically, a woman will wake from sleep to find she is drenched in sweat and has to get up to change her night-clothes, and perhaps even the bedding. Night sweats cause greatly disturbed nights and lack of sleep, for the woman suffering them and perhaps also for her partner who may find himself woken several times in the night as she gets up to wash and change into something dry. Repeated broken nights cause fatigue, loss of concentration, irritability, and a general sense of lethargy.

The underlying cause of a hot flush is a *falling* level of oestrogen. This is not the same as a *low* level: girls before puberty and men have low levels of oestrogen, but they don't suffer hot flushes; women get them when the level of oestrogen in their body has been high and then starts to fall. Women who lose their oestrogen suddenly, as when they have both ovaries removed, tend to get flushes that are particularly troublesome. If the decrease in oestrogen is gradual, the symptoms will be less severe. In most cases, once the body has adjusted to its final low level, the flushes will end.

It is thought that the falling level of oestrogen throws the body's heat-controlling mechanism into confusion, and the 'thermostat' becomes set too low. The result is that the body thinks it is suddenly too hot, so it dilates the blood vessels and sweats to cool itself down. The dilated blood vessels produce redness and a sensation of heat in the skin, but although the skin itself may become several degrees warmer than normal, the body's underlying temperature remains unchanged. Even if the skin hardly becomes warm at all, the woman will still feel hot – usually uncomfortably and embarrassingly so.

Flushes can be triggered by several things – or by nothing. Common causes of a flush are: anxiety, hot weather, moving from a cold room to a hot one, drinking tea, coffee, alcohol or hot drinks, or eating spicy food. However, most flushes don't seem to be triggered by anything. As smoking reduces oestrogen, smokers tend to find flushes more troublesome than non-smokers do.

If you get hot flushes, you may feel freakish, and wonder if everyone is staring at you. In reality, the chances are that no one will notice, and, far from being a freak, 75 per cent of women going through the menopause get hot flushes, just like you. Of that number, 80 per cent still have them a year after they first appeared, 25 per cent still have them five years later, and for an unfortunate 5 per cent, they continue indefinitely.

Hot flushes and night sweats are, therefore, an obvious case for treatment with hormone replacement therapy, and in fact relief from these distressing symptoms is the commonest reason for women wanting to take it. As the problem is caused by falling levels of oestrogen, the flushes cease when these levels are topped up to their normal level. Once oestrogen therapy is started, the situation can be dramatically improved within a few days, and the flushes have usually ceased completely within a few weeks. If you are still troubled with them after three months of therapy, ask your doctor if he will change your dosage of oestrogen; he should be able to find one eventually that relieves your symptoms without causing unpleasant side-effects. Once things have stabilised, the relief will usually continue for as long as you remain on the therapy. However, they may return if you stop the treatment suddenly, move to a hot climate (if you go abroad on holiday, for example), take a course of antibiotics, or come under additional stress. If this happens, ask your doctor's advice.

Taking HRT will eliminate night sweats, dramatically improving the quality of your sleep, and with it your level of fatigue and irritability. Sadly, some general practitioners still prescribe tranquillisers and anti-depressants to women who complain of hot flushes and night sweats, and the insomnia and emotional upsets that they cause. This is difficult to justify, as the problem is due to falling oestrogen, and nothing else. Replace the oestrogen with HRT and the flushes and sweats will disappear, and with them the sleep disturbance they cause and its accompanying fatigue, irritability and lack of wellbeing. If you are on tranquillisers or anti-depressants for these particular menopausal problems, talk to your doctor about the possibility of changing to hormone replacement therapy. (If he 'doesn't believe in it', see page 90 for other suggestions.)

Many women feel they want to 'die of embarrassment' or 'disappear into the floor' when a hot flush strikes them at work or in mixed company. This is largely due to other people's perception of hot flushes; some men and young women may laugh and make unkind remarks. Perhaps we could bring up our sons in such a way that they become men who will not diminish a female colleague's self-esteem at work, but will show kindness and sympathy during what is a very uncomfortable few minutes. Once our daughters know more about the menopause and its causes and effects, perhaps they will help to develop a culture that will ensure attitudes have changed by the time their turn comes.

Flushes have been described as 'something like adolescent acne – an outward sign of natural hormonal changes'. They may be troublesome and embarrassing but (unless you are one of the unfortunate 5 per cent) they do decrease in number and strength, and they will eventually pass as the body adjusts to its lower level of oestrogen. However, just because the menopause is 'natural' doesn't mean you have to put up with its distressing symptoms for months or years, and we are lucky that HRT is now available to relieve them.

Insomnia

Many menopausal women complain of sleep problems. It is difficult to separate sleep problems that are due to low oestrogen from sleep problems that are due to the effects of ageing. If you were previously in good health and your sleep is now disturbed by night sweats, then HRT will almost certainly help. However, if you cannot link your insomnia or other sleep problems to the menopause, then HRT may not help, as the cause is probably not low oestrogen. (You might like to try HRT for, say, two months, and if you still can't sleep after this time, then the insomnia has other causes.) As with hot flushes, some doctors still prescribe tranquillisers and sedatives to women whose sleep disturbance is the result of a deficiency of oestrogen, and this cannot be a good thing. If night sweats are disturbing your sleep, and if as a result of this you feel tired, lethargic, irritable, and find it difficult to concentrate or make decisions, ask your doctor about HRT.

> ❝My problems were that I kept waking in the night drenched through with sweat, or just waking after only 2–3 hours' sleep, and then remaining wide awake for some hours; also I started getting feelings of panic. HRT solved all these problems, although I had to increase the original dose before it really worked. I am now my normal self, and my husband gets a good night's sleep now that I do, so he's happy.❞

Psychological problems and altered moods

❝The psychological problems [of the menopause] tend to be insidious and can impair a woman's ability to control her domestic and work environment . . . They can destroy self-confidence and self-esteem and are an incomprehensible low point in the lives of previously well-adjusted and competent women.❞ from *The Menopause*, J. Studd and M. Whitehead (eds.), 1988.

❝The only word I can use to describe how I felt during this period is wretched. I work in a doctor's surgery and spend my working day in contact with the patients. I was moody, bad-tempered and thoroughly unpleasant to everyone – yet I couldn't stop myself being like that. My feelings about myself reached rock-bottom and my normal self-confidence disappeared completely until I could hardly bring myself to get out of bed in the morning. I think if I'd worked anywhere else I would have lost my job within a few weeks; but luckily the menopause specialist nurse in the practice recognised my changed personality for what it was, suggested I asked my GP about HRT, and I'm now back in the human race again.❞

❝I am the Marketing Director of a large company. As you can imagine, I have a responsible, demanding job, and I need to be on top of it all the time. Before the menopause hit me I was confident, self-assured, full of energy – a real get-up-and-go woman! I couldn't believe that within about six months most of that had gone. Suddenly I was irritable and permanently tired. I dreaded meetings where I would have to make decisions, and my memory became so bad I thought I was going mad. Although part of me resents the fact that so much depends on having the right level of hormones, the rest of me is grateful that at least my falling oestrogen can be topped up with HRT and I'm now just about back to my old self again.❞

If you have had a similar experience, you are not alone. A great many women between the ages of 40 and 60 find they become moody, unable to concentrate, and very tired. Many of the psychological problems of the menopause are due to night sweats causing disturbed sleep, and will resolve themselves once broken nights come to an end. Others are due more directly to the loss of oestrogen. Part of the brain contains many oestrogen receptors, and if oestrogen levels fall, mood changes may occur; once the oestrogen is replaced by HRT, most women find their confidence and self-esteem restored and their problems with mood swings, forgetfulness and anxiety considerably alleviated. HRT is not as reliable in improving these complaints as it is for flushes and sweats, but if your general wellbeing and feelings about yourself have taken a plunge, then it's worth asking about HRT. It won't, however, do anything to alleviate depression, anxiety or unhappiness that existed before the menopause, and which is not due to lowered levels of oestrogen.

Oestrogen seems to have a 'mental tonic' effect, and lowered levels of the hormone during and after the menopause can lead to a whole range of psychological problems, such as:

- less energy and drive
- irritability
- mood changes
- headaches
- feelings of unworthiness
- loss of self-esteem
- loss of self-confidence
- feeling unable to cope

- difficulty in concentrating
- feelings of aggressiveness
- depression
- anxiety
- forgetfulness
- fear of loneliness
- unusually prone to tears
- loss of libido (sex drive)

There are still too many doctors who, faced in the surgery with a woman aged between 40 and 60 complaining about any of these problems, will say, 'I'm afraid it's just your age, my dear,' or 'You'll just have to live with it – there's nothing I can give you that a good night's sleep/doing some voluntary work/joining an evening class won't cure.' And he writes out a prescription for some anti-depressants and hopes she won't bother him again. (In this book, the doctor is depicted as male, simply to avoid confusion with the patient who, in matters concerning the menopause, is inevitably female.)

Prescribing tranquillisers and anti-depressants for problems in the mind that are caused by a fall in oestrogen is difficult to justify. Yet for many women, even nowadays, that is all they get, and then everyone is surprised that it seldom has the desired effect. It is hardly believable that 30–40 per cent of women aged 45–55 with menopausal depression are still prescribed tranquillisers and anti-depressants despite the fact that replacing their oestrogen will usually reduce these symptoms and thereby, in the majority of cases, lift the depression.

Gynaecologist John Studd of King's College, London, has pointed out that there are three times in a woman's life when she is more likely to suffer from depression: before a period, after the birth of a child, and during the menopausal phase of her life (the climacteric). He believes that the massively changing hormone levels at these times are, in part, responsible for these periods of depression. Although many events in a woman's life around the time of the menopause (such as children leaving home, the death or increasing infirmity of elderly parents, and a general awareness of growing older) may all contribute to feelings of depression, men have these worries, too, at this time, yet depression doesn't affect them nearly so much. Depression is twice as common in women as in men, so it would not be surprising to discover that it is often caused by whatever distinguishes a woman from a man, that is her hormones.

The majority of psychiatrists still believe that anti-depressants, tranquillisers or psychotherapy are the best forms of treatment for women at these three critical times of depression, yet they appear to have a low success rate. By contrast, replacing the oestrogen that is probably causing the depression appears to be very effective in many women. If the psychological symptoms are due to a lack of oestrogen, they will respond to a course of HRT; if they are due to some other cause, then HRT will not bring any real benefit. As HRT is a much cheaper form of treatment than psychotherapy or in-patient psychiatric care, it is surely worth considering as a first-line form of treatment for depression that occurs around the time of the menopause.

Changes in the skin

‘What I felt wasn't just ordinary itching. I felt as if insects were crawling around on my skin, especially around my abdomen. I would wake up in the night itching like mad, which was another reason I didn't sleep so well.’

‘An unexpected benefit of HRT has been that my skin has looked so much better. It was beginning to get noticeably thinner, and quite dry and flaky, and that in itself made me suddenly feel about 10 years older – but I'm not trying to look like a film star!’

Improved skin texture is a visible – and welcome – result of taking hormone replacement therapy.

Skin consists of two principal parts: a thin outer layer called the epidermis, and a thicker lower layer called the dermis. Within the dermis is a substance called collagen, and this becomes thinner as oestrogen levels fall, causing the skin as a whole to become thinner. This could be because collagen increases the moisture content of the skin and 'fills it out'. Collagen is lost from the dermis most rapidly in the years immediately after the final period, with up to 30 per cent being lost in the first five years, and about 2 per cent a year after that.

As the thickness of the skin depends on its collagen content, skin condition is related more to the number of years since the menopause than to actual age. Once oestrogen is restored, the collagen starts to increase; where conditions such as thin skin, dry flaky skin, and skin that becomes easily bruised are caused by low oestrogen they are almost always reversible within the first six months of taking HRT. This improvement doesn't continue indefinitely, and balances out after about two years of treatment. However, although skin texture improves significantly, there is no evidence that HRT slows the development of wrinkles!

Not only can good skin improve a woman's self-esteem, it can also be an indication of the state her bones are in. Collagen is also present in bone and, if collagen is being lost visibly from the skin, it is also probably being lost invisibly from the bones. Women with transparent skin are much more likely to have osteoporosis (see Chapter 6) than women with opaque skin. If your skin appears to be getting noticeably thinner, it might be a good idea to talk to your doctor about osteoporosis.

A skin condition that quite a few women suffer from during the early days of the menopause is known as formication. The name comes from the Latin *formica*, meaning 'ant', which aptly describes the feeling you may get of insects crawling just underneath or on top of your skin. It doesn't produce a rash, but the itching can be maddening, and can wake you up in the night. Formication is probably caused by changes in the nerve endings, and the condition can be helped by HRT.

Intermediate symptoms of the menopause

These are symptoms that do not appear until some time after the menopause, but which tend to get more noticeable and troublesome as the years go by:

- bladder problems, such as stress incontinence, and needing to empty the bladder frequently and without warning
- recurrent bacterial infections of the vagina and urethra (the passage through which urine is discharged)
- vaginal dryness
- pain during sexual intercourse
- generalised muscle aches and pains
- thinning skin and hair

Bladder problems and vaginal dryness

These are the most troublesome and common of the inter-
mediate symptoms of the menopause. Vaginal dryness is itself
the cause of pain during sexual intercourse and many of the
recurrent bacterial infections. Without oestrogen, the lining of
the walls of the bladder and urethra shrink and become thinner and drier. They are more likely to crack and split, and
become vulnerable to infection. Within three years of the
menopause, 10–20 per cent of women may visit their doctor
with these problems; amongst women eight years or more
since the menopause, the figure is up to 50 per cent. It may
be embarrassing, but there's a lot of it about. As with hot
flushes, you are not alone, and if only women felt able to talk
about these things more they might feel less isolated in their
discomfort and embarrassment. Surprisingly, few women
realise that these complaints are connected with the
menopause at all. They just think it is all due to getting older
and that nothing can be done about it; but, as with all the
symptoms that are due to lowered levels of oestrogen at the
time of the menopause, something *can* be done about it.

Vaginal dryness and soreness are very common problems
for women in their fifties. The walls of the vagina respond
to the presence of oestrogen, and as the level of the hormone falls, they become thinner and drier and less elastic.
The vagina itself becomes shorter and narrower, and the
cervix secretes less mucus. Noticeable symptoms that result
from this can be dryness, pain during sexual intercourse,
bleeding during intercourse, and a higher risk of bacterial
infections. If HRT replaces the lost oestrogen, the vagina
can be restored to a healthy state, and there is no reason
why you should not continue a fulfilling sex life for as long
as you and your partner want to. (The subject of sex, the
menopause and HRT is discussed fully in Chapter 5.)

Symptoms of pain, discomfort and embarrassment involv-
ing the bladder and urinary tract are felt by a great many
women to be part of the misery of the menopause.

❛I hadn't wet myself since I was a small child. Suddenly one day I coughed fairly violently, and with a horrifying sense of shame and embarrassment, I knew I had done at 55 what I hadn't done since I was about four. Then it started to happen more often, whenever I coughed or laughed or sneezed. At first it was a little trickle, then it became so bad I had to wear sanitary towels most of the time – just in case. A friend of mine who works in a chemist's shop said she knew of many women who bought sanitary towels for this purpose, and who could not bring themselves to buy incontinence pads.❜

The urethra (the canal with carries urine from the bladder to outside your body) is yet another part of you that contains 'oestrogen receptors' and so it responds to the presence of oestrogen by remaining firm, strong and healthy. After the menopause, the walls of the urethra become thinner, more prone to infections like cystitis, and the muscles don't work so well. These changes can cause pain on passing water, and a gradual lessening of bladder control. Complaints such as urgency (needing to pass water with very little warning); frequency (needing to pass water frequently); nocturia (needing to pass water during the night); and stress incontinence (passing urine when you sneeze, cough, laugh or take vigorous exercise), all usually improve significantly after a few weeks of HRT (provided there is no underlying infection or other problem). Up to 30 per cent of post-menopausal women suffer from these complaints, and may need to remain on HRT long-term if the symptoms are not to return.

If you have a continence problem of any sort and don't like to talk to your doctor about it, you may find the surgery has a special Continence Nurse. Her job is to help people achieve continence wherever this is possible, or to manage incontinence if this is inevitable. You will find her helpful and sympathetic, and full of practical suggestions to improve your particular problem, whatever your age.

Other intermediate problems

- Bleeding and shrinking gums sometimes improve with HRT.
- Many women experience ill-defined muscle and joint pains around the time of the menopause, especially in their hands, wrists, elbows, knees, shoulders and lower back. These are often misdiagnosed as arthritis, and this particular type of joint pain usually improves with HRT. Women whose arthritis gets worse around the time of the menopause may find HRT brings some improvement.
- The causes of hair loss and brittle nails are not very well understood; these problems may be linked more to increasing age than to a fall in hormone levels.

Long-term effects of the menopause

While many women are happy to receive treatment for a condition that is bothering them now, far fewer want to take it to prevent something that may (or may not) happen some time in the future. This is a pity, because there are two serious conditions that are directly related to low levels of oestrogen after the menopause: **arterial disease**, which can lead to heart attack and stroke and is often fatal, and **osteoporosis**, which isn't usually directly fatal, but which causes pain, deformity and a considerably reduced quality of life, and can be an indirect cause of death.

Neither of these diseases usually arises until several years after the ovaries have stopped producing oestrogen, but all women are potentially at risk from them the further they get in time from the menopause. The earlier you have the menopause (surgical or natural), the greater the proportion of your life without oestrogen, so the greater your risk of developing arterial disease and osteoporosis, and the more important it is that you are aware of these long-term consequences of low oestrogen and what you can do about it.

This chapter will cover just the role HRT can play in

preventing arterial disease, as osteoporosis is dealt with in Chapter 6.

Arterial disease

Disease of the arteries is the Number One cause of death in women over 50. Whether the cause is heart attack or stroke, arterial disease kills one woman in every four.

The arteries carry blood from the heart all round the body, and so it is important for our health that they remain in good condition. If they become narrowed, or clogged up, then the blood can't flow so freely, and there is a much increased chance that the flow will suddenly become completely restricted, causing a heart attack or a stroke.

Some of the factors that contribute to heart disease are outside our control, such as the natural ageing process, and the hereditary aspect of heart disease; other risk factors we *can* do something about, by giving up smoking, not drinking too much alcohol, taking enough exercise, eating the right diet and learning how to handle stress.

One of the factors that increases the risk of developing diseases of the arteries is being male; until the age of 40–50, far more men than women die of heart disease. In fact, it is unusual for otherwise healthy pre-menopausal women to have heart attacks, whereas, sadly, it is not unusual for men in this age group to do so. The reason is thought to be the protective effect of a woman's oestrogen. Once a woman is past the menopause (whether natural or surgical) her risk of having a heart attack increases, until by the age of 75–80 she has the same risk as men.

The reason for this is possibly to do with cholesterol. There are two forms of cholesterol flowing through the blood vessels: low density lipoproteins (LDLs) which build up on the walls of the blood vessels and are 'bad for you', and high density lipoproteins (HDLs) which are 'good for you' because they latch on to the LDLs and absorb them through the artery walls to be disposed of by other organs in the body. Many years of research have shown that oestrogen lowers the level of LDLs and raises the level of HDLs. As high levels of LDLs increase the risk of arterial disease (by blocking the arteries), and high levels of HDLs are good for you (because they remove the LDLs), oestrogen has a very positive protective effect.

Also, at times of increasing age, when the major arteries of the body are narrowing, HRT is thought to widen them and so allow blood to flow more freely. In fact, women on HRT tend to have healthier arteries than those not on it; even women of 70 or more can benefit from this protective effect of HRT.

As you will read in Chapter 8, there is a small but increased risk of developing breast cancer after several years on HRT, a fact that has received a lot of publicity. However, heart disease and stroke are the largest single cause of death among women in this country, completely dwarfing the number of deaths from breast cancer. The average reader of this book over the age of 50 is many times more likely to die from heart disease or stroke than from breast cancer (although under the age of 50 the risk of breast cancer is greater). A great deal of research has been carried out in recent years into HRT's effect on menopausal symptoms and osteoporosis, but much less into its effect on arterial disease. This balance is beginning to change, and over the next few years more will become known about the effect different hormones have on heart disease and stroke. Although HRT was originally prescribed primarily to treat hot flushes, etc, and more recently also to prevent osteoporosis, it is likely that in future years it will be prescribed mainly for its role in reducing the risk of heart disease and stroke. Even now, it is thought that women who take oestrogen have one-third to one-half the risk of developing these two conditions than women who don't.

(It is worth noting here that almost all the studies that show the beneficial effect of oestrogen on arterial disease have been carried out on women taking oestrogen alone, and not oestrogen with progestogen, although recent work suggests that progestogen may not detract from oestrogen's cardiovascular protection; there have not yet, however, been any results based on long-term data. For more about the disadvantages of progestogen, see the next chapter.)

To gain significant protective effect against arterial disease, you may need to stay on HRT for two years or so, preferably longer, and the effect will diminish once you stop. Even then, the oestrogen only reduces your *risk* of developing these diseases, it cannot guarantee that you won't get them. We are not immortal!

* * *

The first report on the use of hormones to reduce symptoms of the menopause said, in 1935:

> ❛In most patients, symptoms are rather mild, so no treatment is necessary except an instructional and reassuring talk from the medical adviser as to the normality of the symptoms, their temporary nature, the importance of avoiding stress and anxiety, and perhaps the administration of a simple nerve sedative.❜

The writer of this report was right in that these symptoms are all normal, and many of them are temporary. However, that doesn't mean we have to live with them if they are reducing our quality of life. Pain during childbirth or tooth extraction is normal, but most people nowadays would choose to use various methods to reduce it.

If you are one of the lucky ones, and you are not bothered by hot flushes, night sweats, distressing states of mind, vaginal and bladder problems, and if you are at little or no risk of developing osteoporosis, then you will probably feel that HRT would be an unnecessary medical intervention for you.

Few elderly people regard old age as a blessing, yet we all want to get there. To do it, all women have to go through the menopause, with its many and varied symptoms, few of which we would wish upon ourselves if we could redesign female biology from scratch. Women born in this century were the first who could confidently expect to live to three-score-years-and-ten, and most of us will live another 10 or more years beyond that. We want them to be rich, fulfilling years. There is nothing any of us can do to stop the ageing process, but at least many of the problems of the menopause can now be relieved by replacing the oestrogen we all inevitably lose.

Chapter 3

Progestogen – the fly in the ointment

You have probably noticed in life that every silver lining has a cloud! In the case of HRT, the cloud is called progestogen (a synthetic form of the hormone progesterone).

Up to now it has all looked pretty good: whether you have hot flushes, vaginal and bladder problems, mood changes, or even feelings of insects crawling over your skin, replacing oestrogen gives you a good chance of ending these troublesome symptoms of the menopause. HRT even protects you against osteoporosis, and reduces your chance of having a heart attack. It all sounds too good to be true.

If you have had a hysterectomy, you can skip this slightly depressing chapter, because progestogen is not a word that need bother you. But if you still have a uterus (womb) and are considering taking HRT, this chapter is compulsory reading!

In Chapter 1 you read that women produce two hormones as part of the reproductive cycle – oestrogen and progesterone. Thanks to oestrogen, your body maintains itself at a comfortable temperature, your vagina and bladder are in a healthy condition, your skin blooms, your mood lifts, your bones remain strong, and the blood in your arteries flows freely. Oestrogen is what gives you your particularly female characteristics: breasts, broad hips, the distribution of hair, the pitch of your voice; during pregnancy it maintains the lining of the womb and prepares the breasts for the production of milk.

Progesterone is produced in the ovaries after the ovulation phase of the menstrual cycle, and in pregnancy. Its main function is to prepare the womb for a fertilised egg, and to maintain the pregnancy. It also thickens the lining of the womb, reduces secretions from the cervix (the neck of the womb), prevents ovulation, contributes to the retention of water and salt, and works with oestrogen to stimulate milk cells in the breasts. During a menstrual cycle that doesn't result in pregnancy, it is the production of progesterone that contributes to the pre-menstrual feelings of bloatedness, breast tenderness, and general irritability. So although it has an important role to play in the menstrual cycle and pregnancy, progesterone is not exactly an unmixed blessing, and its presence in HRT causes the single most important reason why women who have not had a hysterectomy either don't want this form of treatment at all, or don't stay on it for more than a few months.

To understand why, it is necessary to go back a few decades. In the 1950s and 1960s, oestrogen replacement therapy was used by women in the United States in a big way. By replacing their lost oestrogen they discovered they could be, as the phrase went, 'feminine forever'. At its peak, up to 50 per cent of middle-class American menopausal women were taking oestrogen, often simply so that they would look and feel 20 years younger. Eternal youth and, of course, no more periods. Goodbye old age! Life could now be one long silver lining.

Until up popped that little black cloud. By the 1970s, doctors in the United States had begun to notice a worrying increase in the number of women on oestrogen replacement therapy who developed – and sometimes died of – cancer of the endometrium (the lining of the womb). Suddenly oestrogen therapy was getting a very bad press, and in a short space of time doctors no longer wanted to prescribe it, and women no longer wanted to take it. It seemed as if this wonderful era of eternal youth was over.

Research quickly got under way, and it was discovered

that when a woman took oestrogen on its own the lining of the womb would build up each month and remain there instead being shed as a period in the normal way. Eventually, the lining of the womb would become abnormally thickened, and in some women it became cancerous. The solution was to add a form of the hormone progesterone to the oestrogen therapy every month, so that the lining of the womb did not build up, but was shed each month, as a 'period'. (After the menopause, it is not a true period as it is not triggered by ovulation, nor does it mean you are fertile and could become pregnant; it is an artificial withdrawal bleed, produced when you stop taking each monthly course of progestogen.)

This now seemed the solution to the problem of endometrial cancer and another associated condition called endometrial hyperplasia which is a non-cancerous build-up of the lining of the womb. By taking progestogen with the oestrogen for 10–12 days each month, cancer of the endometrium no longer becomes a risk.

Unfortunately, the snag is now this word 'period'. For most women, the Number One advantage of the menopause is *no more periods*. After 35 years of tampons, sanitary towels, cramps and pre-menstrual tension, this has got to be worth waiting for, and probably worth putting up with flushes, sweats and all the rest for as well.

So you go along to your doctor and he suggests HRT will help your menopausal problems. You agree this seems a good idea, until he says, 'There is one slight drawback: your periods will return'. And he explains how the progestogen part of the HRT is necessary to cause the lining of the womb to come away each month. At this point it's very tempting to ask if you can have your HRT with just the oestrogen, but the answer will be no. Except in very rare cases, if you still have a womb, then you must take progestogen to protect yourself from cancer of the endometrium.

In fact, for most women, the periods will probably not be

too much of a nuisance and will not last forever. As you get older, the lining of the womb will start to atrophy (waste from lack of use), until for a lucky minority the time will come when you no longer have these withdrawal bleeds at all, even if you take progestogen. Until then, the periods will almost certainly be much lighter than before the menopause – often no more than just a little spotting. However, even when these withdrawal bleeds no longer occur, you will still have to take the progestogen, to make sure the lining of the womb does not build up again.

If periods were the end of the problem, you might well feel you could live with it. But, in the same way that progesterone contributes to pre-menstrual tension, bloating and breast tenderness before the menopause, so it may now produce a similar range of symptoms when taken as progestogen in HRT. Towards the end of the 10–12 days in which you take the progestogen, you may get symptoms such as:

- abdominal cramps
- backache
- acne and greasy skin
- headaches
- irritability
- feelings like pre-menstrual tension
- fluid retention, leading to a feeling of bloatedness
- weight gain
- lowered interest in sex
- moodiness

You will see that taking progestogen over-rides several of the advantages of taking oestrogen, causing skin problems, changes in mood, and a decreased interest in sex. It is also possible that it may lessen oestrogen's beneficial effect on heart disease, although some recent research suggests otherwise.

It's therefore understandable that many women who start on an oestrogen and progestogen form of HRT give up after a few months. However, in many cases, these problems diminish after a while. Weight gain is a good example: many women on HRT find they put on several pounds in

the first few months, but the great majority lose most of
what they gain and end up barely a pound or two heavier
than they were originally.

If you find HRT is causing you these sorts of problems,
ask your doctor about changing to a different type of
progestogen. There are different types available, and various
dosages within each type, so there is a good chance you will
eventually find a combination of oestrogen and a progestogen that will give the advantages without the side-effects.
Faced with a woman who has undesirable symptoms at the
first attempt, many doctors still say, 'Well, we've tried
HRT, but it obviously isn't going to work for you. Never
mind', and they just give up, without making any more
attempts at finding an acceptable combination of the two
hormones. If you feel that you need oestrogen (whether to
reduce menopausal symptoms, or to protect yourself from
osteoporosis or artery disease), it would be a great shame if
you gave it up after just a few months.

As you will read in Chapter 4, there are about 20 different combinations in which you can take HRT, so it's highly
likely one of them will be right for you. It just requires a little patience and perseverance from both you and your doctor. Usually, changing to a different progestogen will get rid
of the unwanted side-effects, but if that doesn't work, then
reducing the dosage should work, or possibly taking it for
fewer days each month. However, there is a minimum dose
needed to ensure the lining of the womb is shed each
month, so you shouldn't have too low a dose or for too
short a time. Many women find that vitamin B6 or evening
primrose oil helps reduce unpleasant pre-menstrual symptoms brought on by progestogen.

The good news is that research is being done into new
and better progestogens. Until recently, this hormone could
only be taken in the form of tablets by mouth. As much of
the progestogen gets lost as it passes through the digestive
system, quite a large dose has to be taken so that you end
up with the amount you need, and this large dose is what

causes most side-effects. Progestogen is now also available in a combined progestogen and oestrogen patch (see Chapter 4). It is called Estracombi, and is manufactured by Ciba-Geigy. In this form, the two hormones are absorbed through the skin, and because the digestive system is avoided, a much lower dose can be given to achieve the desired effect, thereby reducing the side-effects. Before long, a completely new generation of progestogens will be available which produce fewer side-effects.

If progestogen in any form really doesn't agree with you, under certain circumstances it may be possible to cut it out altogether. Your doctor would probably only suggest this if you already had osteoporosis and needed to take oestrogen but were finding the side-effects of progestogen so intolerable that you had to give up. The big disadvantage of doing this, however, is that you would have a small but definite risk of developing cancer or other disorders of the lining of the womb. You would need careful counselling about this, and your doctor would probably suggest that every one to two years you had a biopsy: a small piece of the lining of the womb would be removed and sent for examination to see whether there was any sign of cancer or other disorders. Nowadays, for women who have osteoporosis of the spine but who really cannot take progestogen, a new non-hormone drug called etidronate might be the solution (see page 76).

If it is the 'withdrawal bleed' that is putting you off HRT, there is a third alternative, known as 'no-bleed HRT' (because the aim of it is that it should eliminate distressing menopausal symptoms without producing periods), or 'continuous/combined HRT' (because you take combined oestrogen and progestogen continuously). No-bleed HRT involves taking a small dose of progestogen *every* day, instead of for just 10–12 days a month. The theory is that this method eventually leads to amenorrhoea (a complete absence of periods).

A new form of no-bleed HRT called tibolone (marketed by Organon Laboratories under the brand name of Livial) combines the properties of oestrogens, progestogens and androgens in a single tablet taken daily, and has proved effective in the treatment of hot flushes, night sweats and headaches. Although it is similar to oestrogen, it does not stimulate the lining of the womb, so withdrawal bleeds don't occur, in theory at least; in fact many women do continue to have regular bleeds for several months, but in most cases they eventually cease. About 20 per cent of women also get irregular bleeding between periods for many months, which is not really acceptable. In theory, this seems a form of HRT that will eventually combine no periods with reducing hot flushes and night sweats, and which has few side-effects. Short-term research data shows it offers protection against osteoporosis, but no long-term data is available yet. Nor is it known what the effects might be of taking progestogen every day instead of for 10–12 days a month, and as yet there is no research information on whether Livial gives the same benefits to the heart as other types of oestrogen therapy do. More research is needed, but it could be the form of HRT that women are looking for. (See also page 50.) Other pharmaceutical companies are also developing forms of HRT which do not produce a monthly bleed, and some of these should be available soon, including at least one (Kliogest, by Novo Nordisk Pharmaceuticals) which is expected to be licensed for osteoporosis.

The other disadvantage of progestogen is that it may negate some of the advantages of oestrogen in preventing disease of the arteries. Oestrogen appears to reduce fats and cholesterols that circulate in the blood, and progestogen may increase them. So, as long as you need to take progestogen, you might not be getting the lowered risk of heart attack and stroke that you would get from oestrogen on its own. Encouraging news is that the newer forms of progestogens have only minor effects on blood fats.

By contrast, small quantities of progestogen help to prevent osteoporosis. There is also a possibility that it might slightly decrease your chance of developing breast cancer, but as some research has suggested otherwise it is difficult to be sure. The relationship between breast cancer and HRT is discussed in Chapter 8.

In conclusion, if you still have a uterus, the form of HRT you take must contain a progestogen, but with any luck the new non-oral low-dose varieties will reduce the side-effects, new progestogens may overcome many of the present disadvantages, and the future of no-bleed HRT looks hopeful.

　One of the most urgent requirements for successful HRT would seem to be the development of better progestogens, and better ways of administering them. from *The Change – Women, Ageing and the Menopause*, Germaine Greer, 1991.

Chapter 4

Pills, patches and implants – How to take HRT

'For oestrogen replacement therapy to become universally acceptable, it is essential that we provide the most effective type of treatment with the least side effects.' from *The Menopause*, J. Studd and M. Whitehead (eds.), 1988.

Women vary enormously in their response to different medications, so what is 'the most effective type of treatment with the least side effects' for one woman may be an ineffective type with bad side-effects for another. Fortunately, there are over 20 different ways in which oestrogens and progestogens can be combined into hormone replacement therapy, so with your doctor's help you should be able to find one that is right for you.

However, there are two factors that may prevent you ever getting that far: one is that the initial side-effects put you off the whole idea of HRT and you decide just to give up without trying different types; the other is that your doctor may be unable or unwilling to suggest alternatives for you. With the best will in the world, no doctor is able to remember every variety of every form of treatment that is available for all his patients, so he has his 'favourites' that he uses most of the time because he knows they work well. If one of them doesn't work, he then has to start referring to the various publications that list different forms of treatment, and just hope that the one he chooses is the right one for that particular patient. Usually, when the average general practitioner suggests that HRT may be the answer to your menopausal problems, he will almost certainly prescribe his 'favourite' preparation because his experience has shown it to work with most of his patients. It may well work for you, or it may not. It may relieve your symptoms without producing side-effects, or it may not. However, if this one doesn't help, another one probably will.

The number and types of HRT preparations available have increased enormously in the last 10 years, and are still increasing each year. Those most commonly used in the UK are in the form of tablets, patches and implants, all available in different strengths. Less commonly used here, but varying in popularity in other countries, are creams, gels, pessaries, suppositories and injections.

Some preparations come as combined 'calendar packs' of oestrogen and progestogen, others come with each hormone packed singly. If you are taking a combined pack, and can't get the balance of oestrogen and progestogen right to give relief of symptoms without side-effects, your doctor can prescribe the hormones separately to get the right dosage of each. Both hormones are available in different strengths from different pharmaceutical companies, which allows great flexibility and should make it possible for you and your doctor to get it right.

With the exception of implants, any treatment can be stopped at any time, or the dosage can quickly be adjusted, but you will probably get a return of menopausal symptoms if you stop suddenly. (More about this later in the chapter.)

The first decision you and your doctor will make is whether HRT is suitable for you at all. (Reasons why you may not be able to take it are discussed in Chapter 7.) The next thing to consider is whether you take HRT in an oral form, that is as tablets, or whether a non-oral route (patch, implant or cream) would be better.

Oral HRT – tablets taken by mouth

This is the form most usually prescribed by doctors, especially to women who are starting on HRT, but it isn't always necessarily the best. It has the advantage that it is easy to take, can be stopped at any time, and is cheaper than other forms. The main disadvantage is that the tablet has to contain a fairly high dose of hormone because between 30 per cent and 80 per cent may be lost as it passes through the digestive system before it gets into the blood supply and starts to work. The hormone also has to pass through the liver, where it can cause other problems. It is this comparatively high dose compared to other methods that can cause many of the side-effects. (Even so, oral HRT contains only about the same level of hormone as the body produces naturally before the menopause, and a dose many times lower than is in the contraceptive pill.) Another disadvantage is what the doctor calls 'compliance', that is he has no way of knowing that you really are taking the tablets every day.

Although the great majority of women on oral HRT get on with it very well, some find it a nuisance to have to remember to take a pill every day; others feel it is a daily reminder that they are taking a form of medication they might believe is 'unnatural'. If you think these feelings might concern you, you might be happier with an implant (see page 44).

Being able to stop the therapy suddenly is a big advantage when you first start, and this is one reason why most doctors start their patients on oral HRT. The most commonly prescribed oral HRT is Prempak-C, with Cyclo-Progynova (and its revised version, Nuvelle) and Trisequens a much lower second and third choice (all contain oestrogen and progestogen tablets). Of oral oestrogen without progestogen (for women who have had a hysterectomy), the commonest is Premarin, then Progynova.

HRT by mouth may be an unsuitable first choice (as

compared with non-oral methods such as the patch and the implant) for those who have or have had liver trouble, high blood pressure, chronic digestive disorders (including gall-bladder disease) or a history of blood clotting.

If after a good trial of HRT tablets you are still bothered by undesirable side-effects, ask your doctor about lowering the dose, or changing to a patch, an implant or a cream. If your menopausal symptoms are not being relieved adequately, a higher dose may be necessary.

Many women ask, 'What happens if I miss one or two tablets?' Unlike the contraceptive pill, this is not really a problem. After all, HRT is not a contraceptive, and women past the menopause can no longer become pregnant, even those who have a breakthrough bleed each month induced by the progestogen. The only effect of missing one or more tablets is that you might get breakthrough bleeding at an unexpected time; if you miss several tablets you will probably get a return of hot flushes and other symptoms until you start taking them again.

Transdermal HRT – the patch

The patch is a circular piece of 'plaster' that you stick on to a fleshy part of you. In the centre is a reservoir of oestrogen that is carried through the surface of your skin in a base of alcohol.

Probably the biggest advantage the patch has over tablets is that, because the oestrogen is absorbed through the skin (doctors call this 'transdermal' HRT, meaning 'across the skin') and does not have to go through the liver and the rest of the digestive system, it is taken in a much lower dose and has fewer side-effects. It is easy to use, and easy to stop if you find it doesn't agree with you. Also, the oestrogen is absorbed at a slow, constant rate, whereas if you use oral HRT you are taking the hormone in one dose all at once, which can increase the likelihood of side-effects, particularly in the digestive system.

The patch is simple to use: you just stick it on to a well-padded area of clean, dry skin, such as the buttocks, abdomen or upper thighs, and change to a new patch every 3–4 days, by which time all the alcohol and oestrogen will have been absorbed. You must not stick it on to the breasts. The main drawback with this form of HRT is that about one-third of women find they develop red and itchy skin at the site of the patch, and in a very small percentage this becomes so severe that they have to give up. This is caused by the alcohol contained in the patch and there are two possible solutions. One is to move the patch to a new area of skin every day (but still only having a new patch every 3–4 days), and sticking it down with a piece of elastoplast across it. The other is to wave the patch about in the air for a few seconds before applying it so that some of the alcohol evaporates. Don't do this for too long, however, as it is the alcohol that transports the oestrogen through the skin; no alcohol means no oestrogen. More of the oestrogen is absorbed through the abdomen than through the buttocks or upper thigh, but the buttocks usually give the least skin irritation. (Before long, a new HRT patch will be available without an alcohol base; this should eliminate the problem of skin irritation.)

The skin reacts more to the patch in a hot, humid climate, so some women find it a problem if they go to a hot country on holiday. Leaving the patch off when you lie in the sun is one solution, or possibly changing to tablet HRT while you are away, but this might cause undesirable side-effects. If the patch comes off after swimming or a bath or shower, just stick the same patch back on again with some elastoplast.

The patch comes in three different strengths: 25, 50 and 100 micrograms of a form of oestrogen called oestradiol. If you find it is not having the desired effect, don't be tempted to change to a new patch more frequently as this will not increase the amount of oestrogen you absorb. If you are not happy with its effect, ask your doctor about changing to a patch with a higher or lower dose.

The patch is generally well tolerated, and many prefer it to tablets and are less likely to give up. As before, if you haven't had a hysterectomy, you will have to take progestogen for 10–12 days a month. Until fairly recently, progestogen was only available in tablet form, but there is now a combined oestrogen and progestogen patch called Estracombi, manufactured by Ciba-Geigy. For the first two weeks of the cycle, oestrogen-only patches are worn for 3–4 days each; for the following two weeks, the double oestrogen and progestogen patches are worn for 3–4 days each. Because each double patch contains both hormones, it is not possible to use only the oestrogen patch for this phase of the cycle and to leave the progestogen patch in its box! The manufacturers report that symptoms similar to premenstrual syndrome may be a problem for up to three months, but these should diminish after that time.

The patch method of taking HRT has the same beneficial effects as oral HRT on hot flushes, night sweats, disturbed sleep, changing moods and vaginal dryness. Research suggests that, except at the lowest doses, it also preserves bone in 85–95 per cent of women, but because it is a comparatively new form of HRT it is not yet known for certain the extent to which it provides the same protection against arterial disease. Like oral HRT, the patch can cause breast tenderness, spotting, bloating and feelings of nausea, but these are seldom severe.

Subcutaneous HRT – the implant

'Subcutaneous' means 'beneath the skin', and this is how the implant works. A tiny pellet, about the size of the tip of a lead pencil, is inserted under the skin of the lower abdomen. The technique is simple, takes about 5 minutes, and can often be carried out in a general practitioner's surgery under a local anaesthetic, leaving little or no mark.

The big advantage of an implant is that, once it has been

inserted, you can forget about it for several months. No need to take tablets or change patches. Unlike other forms of HRT, it can also be combined with small quantities of the hormone testosterone if your doctor thinks this would help you. Although testosterone is the male hormone, it is also produced in the ovaries of women, so it is not unnatural to receive it. It can be helpful for women who have certain psycho-sexual problems, a drop in libido (interest in sex), much reduced energy levels or severe loss of confidence. Being a male hormone, it may cause a slight increase in facial hair.

Nearly all women with implants gain relief from hot flushes, and three-quarters gain relief from depression. Improved collagen levels lead to better skin and stronger bones.

As with the patch, the oestrogen is released straight into the bloodstream, and avoids the digestive system, so a lower dose can be used, giving fewer side-effects than oral HRT. There is no question of forgetting to take it, or of suffering the skin irritation some women get with the patch. It also avoids the necessity of 'popping a pill every day', which is what many women don't like about HRT; until it needs replacing you can forget you are using it at all. It also offers good protection against osteoporosis, except at the lowest dosage.

The implant does not last forever, and it will need to be replaced every 4–6 months, depending on when the level of oestrogen in the implant falls and the menopausal symptoms return. You will need to return to your GP or gynaecologist for a replacement. Although this may seem rather a nuisance, it does ensure that you are regularly monitored, and a check-up may also detect irregularities that might otherwise have gone unnoticed.

The implant certainly has several advantages, especially over oral HRT. It does, however, have some disadvantages: A small minority of women find that their menopausal symptoms recur at ever-shorter intervals, so that they appear to need the implant replacing after, say, five months to begin with, then after four months, then three and so on. When they are tested, it is found that they have levels of oestrogen that are not only normal, but often much higher than normal, yet they are still suffering from problems, such as hot flushes and depression, caused by low or falling oestrogen. Along with symptoms of oestrogen deficiency, some women may also get symptoms of too much oestrogen, such as breast tenderness, nausea and bloating. It is a conundrum, and research into why this happens is still continuing.

This condition is called tachyphylaxis, and has received unfavourable publicity following reports of some recent research into it. One or two newspapers decided that it suggested the women were 'addicted' to oestrogen, because they needed ever-higher doses at ever-more-frequent intervals. This type of reporting is irresponsible and unjustified, but many newspapers seem unwilling to present HRT in a neutral light, choosing either to extol its 'sexy forever' image or to condemn it for exaggerated side-effects.

The problem of tachyphylaxis should not, however, be dismissed as irrelevant, because for the small minority of women affected by it, it can be a serious disadvantage, and one for which doctors can't at present agree on a solution. Simply to refuse further HRT in any form produces a return of the symptoms and much suffering; it may also be a dangerous approach in women whose falling oestrogen is producing feelings of depression. However, to replace the implant at ever-closer intervals in a woman whose oestrogen level may be well above normal is not desirable either. It is obviously an area in which more research is needed. If you feel you are developing this condition, talk to your doctor about a gradual withdrawal from this type of HRT, as a different type might be the solution for you. He may decide to monitor your blood oestradiol level regularly, and to replace the implant when it falls to a certain level.

The second disadvantage of the implant concerns those women who still have a uterus and who need to take progestogen. The raised levels of oestrogen from an implant are eliminated from the body only very slowly, so that even once you have stopped using implants the lining of the womb continues to thicken every month and you need to continue taking progestogen until this stops happening. Unfortunately, this thickening of the lining of the womb can continue for up to three or four years after the final implant has been removed, so progestogen needs to be taken all this time to avoid the risk of endometrial cancer. Once the progestogen no longer produces a withdrawal bleed, then you can stop taking it, but there is no fixed time limit on this – it depends on how your body works. It may be only a few months, but it may be much longer.

Like the patch, the implant releases its oestrogen slowly, so it produces fewer side-effects. Unlike the patch, however, if it doesn't agree with you it is very difficult to remove it, so you may just have to put up with it until its effect wears off. For this reason, many doctors do not suggest an implant until a woman has already tried HRT in other forms. It is particularly suitable for women who have had a hysterectomy, as they have no need to take progestogen. Some gynaecologists will insert the implant at the end of the hysterectomy operation if this is what you feel you would like.

Implants come in three different strengths (25, 50 and 100 milligrams); the higher dose lasts longer, and continues to relieve severe symptoms longer.

Percutaneous HRT – creams and gels

For women several years past the menopause, one of the most troublesome symptoms of low oestrogen is 'atrophy of the vaginal and urogenital tract'. To put it another way, the vagina becomes so dry that sex becomes difficult, continence problems develop, and infections occur in the vagina and urethra. One medical dictionary defines atrophy as 'wasting away, from disuse or lack of nutrition'. In the case of the vagina and urethra, the atrophy is caused by a lack of the 'nutrition' of oestrogen.

It is a problem that tends to get more noticeable as the years go by, affecting mainly women from their fifties onwards, and for many of them it will be the first time they have needed to see the doctor about menopausal symptoms. Perhaps our typical woman 'sailed through the menopause', or lived with it without too many problems, but now she finds that a dry vagina means that sex is becoming painful, and she is starting to notice embarrassing 'dribbles' of urine.

This is the point at which she should *not* think, 'Oh, I'm just getting older, there's nothing that can be done about it.' There is, and it's called HRT.

❝Sex started to be uncomfortable, and I thought it was just my age, even though I was only 49. It never occurred to me that this might be a symptom of the menopause, or that anything could be done about it. In any case, I wouldn't have wanted to talk to my doctor about something so personal. Eventually I plucked up courage to see the Practice Nurse at the surgery, and she was very helpful. I didn't want to take HRT as it seems unnatural, but I now use just a vaginal oestrogen cream, and it has made all the difference.❞

As well as being available as tablets, patches and implants, oestrogen can also be applied as a cream. Used in the vagina, it makes the lining thicker, moist and healthy, less vulnerable to infection and more open to stimulation during sexual intercourse. The cream is especially suitable for vaginal dryness, soreness, discharge, pain during sexual intercourse, and vaginitis, and it can be very helpful for some bladder and continence problems. When you first start using oestrogen cream, you may need a fairly high dose, as absorption through the walls of the vagina is usually poor, especially in cases of vaginitis. Once the walls revert to their previous healthy state, however, absorption of the cream will be higher, so a low regular dose should be sufficient, minimising side-effects.

The cream is absorbed through the walls of the vagina into the bloodstream, so it would not be suitable for women who should not take any form of HRT (see Chapter 7). Also, because it contains only a low level of oestrogen, it is not particularly effective for treating hot flushes, nor does it give protection against osteoporosis. It is also important to be aware that it is a *treatment* for vaginal dryness, not a lubrication, so it shouldn't be used just before sexual intercourse. If you do use it then, your partner could absorb undesirably high levels of oestrogen, and may even, in extreme cases, experience some breast enlargement!

If you have not had a hysterectomy, you may be advised to use the cream for a few months only, then your doctor will review it and see whether you need to be taking progestogen. In many cases, use of the cream form of HRT does not give a high enough level of oestrogen to thicken the lining of the womb or necessitate taking progestogen, so it is a particularly suitable form of replacement therapy for older women who do not want the return of periods or need treatment for hot flushes, and whose only menopausal problems are vaginal and some loss of continence.

Vaginal oestrogen is also available as a pessary, called Vagifem (manufactured by Novo Nordisk Pharmaceuticals), that is inserted high up into the vagina with a special applicator. It works in the same way, and for the same conditions, as a vaginal cream.

In some countries (such as France), oestrogen is available as a gel as an alternative to the tablet, patch or implant. Unlike the vaginal creams available in the UK, the gel contains enough oestrogen to eliminate menopausal symptoms such as hot flushes. It is rubbed into the skin of the abdomen or thighs, and French women find it more acceptable than HRT in tablet or patch form. Perhaps it may become available in the UK if enough women press hard enough for the range of HRTs to be extended.

Continuous/combined HRT

As mentioned on page 36, this is a new form of 'no-bleed' HRT produced in response to the high drop-out rate among women who have not had a hysterectomy and who don't want to have regular withdrawal bleeds. Although there has not yet been very much published data on it, it is increasingly being prescribed in the expectation that women will be willing to stay on HRT for longer. Different brands should be available soon. The brand currently available is Livial, and the manufacturers, Organon, describe it as having 'combined progestogenic, oestrogenic and androgenic properties', that is, it works in the same way as progestogens, oestrogens and androgens work. By taking a combination of these hormones in tablet form on a continuous basis (rather than by taking progestogen for just 10–12 days each month), it is hoped that eventually bleeds will stop, though this may take up to a year, doesn't work in all cases, and can produce irregular bleeding in the meantime. (If you continue to get a withdrawal bleed on 'no-bleed' HRT, your doctor may feel it is appropriate to prescribe a one-off dose of progestogen to clear the lining of the uterus, which should prevent further bleeds.) This type of HRT helps mood changes and loss of libido, as well as other symptoms of the menopause. More long-term research is needed before its effectiveness against osteoporosis is known for certain, but a 'no-bleed HRT' is definitely a step in the right direction. If you would like to take HRT for its benefits, but really cannot face the return of monthly 'periods', why not ask your doctor about this new form? It is only recommended for women at least 12 months past their final period.

Getting the dosage right

There is such a wide range of dosages available that your doctor should be able to adjust your prescribed dose to your symptoms. If your symptoms are mild, you will start on a low dose; if they are severe you will start on a higher dose. (The further you are from the menopause, the more likely you are to get side-effects in the early days of taking oestrogen, so a low dose would probably be prescribed for you initially.) If the low dose is not getting rid of the symptoms, ask your doctor if he can give you a higher dose; if the higher dose is producing unpleasant side-effects, ask for a lower dose. Women who have had a hysterectomy or oophorectomy will usually be started on a higher dose, as their symptoms will probably be more severe than women passing through a natural menopause.

If you have severe symptoms of breast tenderness, nipple sensitivity, leg cramps, continuing weight gain and feelings of nausea, you might feel better on a lower dose of oestrogen. If you develop acne, bloatedness, disturbances of your digestive system, a drop in libido, breast discomfort, and feelings of pre-menstrual irritability, then you might feel better on a lower dose of progestogen. However, before you rush off to the doctor, be prepared to stick with your initial treatment for two or three months, unless the HRT is giving you really awful side-effects; in most cases they diminish considerably, and often go completely after a few months.

Women who start HRT before their periods stop completely may find it takes longer to get the dosage exactly right. This is because if you are still having natural periods, then you are still producing some oestrogen, even though its falling levels may be causing hot flushes, night sweats and all the rest. If you take extra oestrogen in the form of HRT, don't be surprised if you suffer some of the effects of this extra dose. Also, as your own level of oestrogen falls steadily, your HRT dose may need gradually to be increased in order to compensate.

The other group of women who may initially suffer side-effects from higher doses of oestrogen (tender breasts, for example) are those who are many years past the menopause and haven't produced much oestrogen of their own for a very long time. If this happens to you, your doctor may suggest that you start on a lower dose, and then progress to a higher dose when your body has adjusted to the oestrogen. Alternatively, it may help if you take the HRT on alternate days to start with. You may also find that evening primrose capsules bring relief for breast tenderness.

As well as adjusting the dosage to menopausal symptoms, your doctor will want to consider whether you are at risk of osteoporosis or arterial disease. If you are, he will probably suggest starting at a medium or high dose, as the low dose may not give enough protection for some women.

When should I start taking HRT, and how long should I stay on it?

The answer to these questions is, 'It depends on your symptoms'. **If you are not bothered by menopausal symptoms**, nor at risk of developing osteoporosis or arterial disease, then don't feel pressured by your friends, family or the media to take it. You do not need it, and to take it would be an unnecessary medical intervention. Despite what the papers say, it will not keep you 'young and sexy forever', and if this is why you want to take it perhaps you should look carefully at yourself, your relationships and your underlying fears.

If, however, you are being bothered by hot flushes, night sweats, and the various early signs of the menopause, then you might want to start HRT as soon as these signs start having a negative effect on your life. This may well be while you are still having periods, but you can still start HRT, although it may be difficult to get the level of treatment exactly right.

Although you may accept all this, some women find the higher rate of side-effects and the irregular bleeds put them off HRT completely and they are then reluctant to consider it again in a few years' time when different symptoms occur. If you have been put off HRT for this reason, you may find that, in the meantime, new forms of HRT have become available that would reduce the problem. Again, talk to your doctor about this.

If you are under about 45 and have just had a hysterectomy, and especially if you have just had an oophorectomy, you will probably be prescribed HRT straight away to overcome possibly quite severe menopausal symptoms. Don't be tempted to give up after a few weeks or months, because your risk of developing osteoporosis is higher than average. If HRT doesn't seem to agree with you, ask your doctor about changing the dosage, or about changing to a different type. Unfortunately, many doctors suggest that women with an early menopause (surgical or natural) use HRT for only a few months to help hot flushes, etc, and do not mention the long-term need to prevent osteoporosis and arterial disease. A survey of members of the National Osteoporosis Society discovered that less than 2 per cent of sufferers who had had a hysterectomy or oophorectomy in the past had been offered treatment with HRT; it is highly likely that if they had been able to receive HRT during the years immediately after the operation they would not be suffering from osteoporosis now.

If you are some years past the menopause you may be being troubled by vaginal and continence problems, so this is a good time to consider HRT to overcome these tiresome and embarrassing consequences of the menopause. You can start now, regardless of whether you ever took it in earlier years.' If you tried it some years ago and didn't get on with it, you may find that one of the newer preparations will suit you better. If, in the meantime, you have had a hysterectomy, you will no longer need to take progestogen.

If you are at risk of developing osteoporosis you
should start within about five years of the menopause for
maximum effect, as these are the years of greatest bone loss;
catch it then and your risks of a fractured hip or vertebra of
the spine are greatly reduced. However, even starting much
later will still give some benefit, and there are plenty of
women who start after the age of 70 and still gain great
benefit. There really is no time at which you are too old to
start.

Much more research is needed into the effectiveness of
HRT in older women, as most doctors in the UK seem
reluctant to prescribe it to a woman over 65. This is a pity,
as it can be of great benefit to them. The risk of developing
osteoporosis and heart disease is much greater over the age
of 65, so this would seem a good time of life to be taking
HRT. Obviously, women with a uterus do not like the idea
of returning to a monthly bleed, which may be heavy or
painful, and they may also experience breast tenderness and
leg cramps. An increase in sexuality can be quite disturbing
after several years without it. This is balanced against an
increased sense of wellbeing, less stiffness in joints and muscles, and more energy. Once again, it is a question of bal-
ancing the advantages to you against the disadvantages, and
when no-bleed HRT is in general use this may greatly
affect how older women feel about it.

How long you stay on HRT will depend on you, your
symptoms and your long-term risks. For most women, two
years is about average for hot flushes, etc, but if they return
when you stop the HRT, then you will probably want to
keep it on for a while longer. You may be one of those
women who need HRT for five years, or even much longer,
to keep flushes at bay.

For relief of vaginal dryness, vaginitis and recurrent vaginal infections, you will probably want to stay on HRT for
as long as you choose to remain sexually active. Sex doesn't
have to stop in your fifties! For conditions which simply
become worse as the years go by, such as incontinence,

osteoporosis and arterial disease, you may decide to stay on
HRT for years, perhaps for the whole of your life (but see
Chapter 7 about the connection between long-term HRT
and a slightly increased risk of breast cancer). If you don't
like the idea of taking it for so long, it is thought that even
five years' treatment in the years immediately after the
menopause will considerably reduce your chances of an
osteoporotic fracture.

In the end, you will continue for as long as the benefits
to you appear to outweigh the disadvantages or risks. Sadly,
the majority of women stop taking HRT after about six
months, perhaps because of side-effects, or a return of
monthly periods, or because of scare stories in the media. In
reality, there is no reason why most women should not be
able to remain on it indefinitely. Should you develop conditions such as a coronary thrombosis, blood clotting, gallbladder disease, cancer of the breast or uterus or ovary,
liver or kidney disease, or if you have a big operation like a
hip replacement, your doctor will probably advise you to
stop taking it. Some doctors, however, feel HRT may safely
be continued even in these circumstances, especially if coming off it might reduce your quality of life significantly more
than suffering these various other diseases would. As with
everything medical, in the end when you start taking HRT,
and how long you remain on it, should be a joint decision
made between you and your doctor.

How do I stop taking HRT?

When you decide you want to stop taking HRT, ask your
doctor about reducing the dosage gradually, as this will prevent a return of short-term symptoms, like hot flushes. A
possible routine might be: If you are taking HRT as tablets,
change to a lower dose tablet for a few weeks, then take
one every alternate day for a few weeks, then just once or
twice a week for two weeks, then stop altogether. If you are
using a patch, change to a lower dose patch for a few

weeks, then leave 1–2 days between changing patches without using one at all, then leave 3–4 days between patches, then, after you have been wearing a patch for only half the time, you should be able to stop.

Implants are more difficult to cut down on, so talk to your doctor about this. He may suggest that when your current implant comes to an end you try tablets or patches that are easier to cut down.

During this 'weaning off' process, some symptoms may return, but they will probably not be frequent or severe. If they are, you will have to decide whether to live with the symptoms or go back to full-time HRT. Flushes and night sweats are usually worse in hot weather or when you are under stress, so it is easier to stop taking HRT when the weather is cooler and when you are feeling calm and in control of your life.

What happens when I stop taking HRT?

Once your body is no longer receiving the replacement oestrogen, the symptoms of oestrogen deficiency will start to return. For hot flushes, unless you are several years past the menopause (or have been cutting down gradually), you will probably notice them appear within a few days; but you will continue to have the benefit of oestrogen on the condition of your skin, bones, vagina and bladder for a few months after you stop. Eventually, however, your skin will become thinner, your vagina drier, your bones less dense, and bladder problems may return.

Nature has pre-determined for you how long your hot flushes and other short-term symptoms will last, and taking HRT will not affect this. So, for example, if you were genetically destined to have flushes for two years and you stop HRT after eighteen months, then the flushes will last for another six months; if you stop HRT after two and a half years, you will probably get some flushes as your body's level of oestrogen falls, but once you have stopped taking it and oestrogen levels have stabilised again, the flushes should stop. What you can't know, however, is what timespan Nature has in mind for you, so it is impossible to predict exactly how you will be affected by the withdrawal of replacement oestrogen.

Chapter 5

Sex and sexuality at the menopause

‹WOMEN TAKE HRT TO REMAIN SEXY FOREVER›

‹HUSBANDS CAN'T KEEP UP WITH NYMPHO WIVES ON HRT›

‹FIFTY PLUS? NOW YOU CAN LOOK THIRTY AGAIN›

Depending on what newspapers and magazines you read, you might have seen headlines like those above. Certain parts of the press seem obsessed with the idea that taking HRT is about nothing more than having the looks and sexuality of a TV star. Every year, dozens of interviews are conducted with television and screen personalities who are now in their fifties and sixties 'and look twenty years younger'.

In some ways, this can be a thoroughly good thing. For too many centuries, the older woman has been neglected, and treated as almost invisible. As far as The Real World is concerned, she just doesn't exist. Newspapers and magazines seldom feature older women in their own right; if they are mentioned at all it is usually as the wife or mother of a man who is making the news. Books end when the beautiful heroine marries the hero; sometimes the story extends to the years of bringing up children, but how many novels can you think of in which the principal character is a woman of

50 or 60? It has been said that 'Sensitive treatment of the ageing woman . . . is not a dominant theme in Anglo-American literature.' Too true! Once you are past child-bearing years it is almost as if you move, in one swift step, to being an unimportant old crone.

Now all this is changing, and HRT can take some of the credit. Suddenly many older women look and feel younger. They don't mind giving their age, because it provokes the response, 'Goodness, are you really? You don't look a day over 45,' and that makes them feel good. Well, it would, wouldn't it? Being more energetic, more confident and still looking youngish, they are visible once more, and that has got to be a good thing. Good for the individual woman and her own self-esteem, and good for womankind in general.

However, this book will not be plugging hormone replacement as an elixir for eternal youth. You will not read in these pages that you, too, can be a sex-kitten forever. If your husband is glancing sideways at younger women, your elderly parents are driving you mad, and your daughter looks how you would like to look, HRT will not magically put your world to rights. It may help mend a breaking marriage, or increase your sex drive, or make you feel 10 years younger, or it may not do any of these things. But it *will* make you feel better able to cope with what the world is throwing at you, and give you a better feeling about yourself.

One of the problems of the 'sex kitten' image is that it actually puts many women off taking HRT. Or they become reluctant to tell their friends they are on it in case they get comments like, 'Oh, is your husband going off with someone else?', as if the only reason a woman takes HRT is to keep her husband in her bed. And many doctors wonder if a woman is enquiring about taking it just so that she can remain 'youthful'. Yes, there *are* reasons why it can help you maintain a satisfying sex life for many years but, as you will have read so far, it has many other advantages, too, and to concentrate on the Eternal Youth image is to trivialise HRT and to diminish women.

ᏀAfter I am waxed old shall I have pleasure, my lord being old also?Ꮔ Sarah (wife of Abraham) in Genesis 18:12.

ᏀI finally plucked up courage to see my doctor. He seemed surprised that a woman of my age (I'm 53 and happily married) should be reluctant to stop having sexual intercourse. He made me feel a freak, the female equivalent of a Dirty Old Man.Ꮔ

The menopause is thought of by many (especially by men and by younger women) as 'the beginning of the end', a time of decline and degeneration, especially sexually. But it needn't be like that. The end of fertility doesn't mean the end of sexuality, let alone the end of femininity. With 30 years or so left, that's just as well! The woman reaching the menopause now is unlikely to view this time as the end of her sexual years, and nor should her doctor, nor society in general. If she has sexual difficulties, they should not be pushed aside.

Many men and women are reluctant to talk to their GPs about sexual problems, as he is quite likely to dismiss it as an unimportant matter in older people. The average young doctor might be quite surprised that a couple in their sixties should still be having an enjoyable sex life, and wanting to continue for many more years. Even couples in their fifties are often considered 'over the hill as far as all that sort of thing is concerned'.

As you have read at various points in this book, one of the symptoms of the menopause is vaginal dryness. Reduced levels of oestrogen diminish the sexual response and cause the cervix to secrete less mucus, so the vagina becomes dry, intercourse is more painful, and you get less pleasure from it. You lose interest in sex, and therefore have sexual intercourse less often. And because you have it less often, less mucus is produced so the vagina becomes drier, and a vicious circle is set up: dry vagina, painful intercourse, less pleasure, less sex, less mucus secretion, drier vagina. This is something that can start at any time around the menopause, and becomes steadily more noticeable as the years pass. It is by replacing the oestrogen and increasing vaginal lubrication that HRT probably has its main effect on renewing sexual enjoyment, and for many women the oestrogen can also – but not always – top up a falling libido at this time.

Loss of libido

This has many causes, and is not only experienced by women. The level of sexual interest starts to fall, and then continues to decline, in men and women in their middle years. While some women undoubtedly find HRT of tremendous benefit to their sexual lives, others find it little or no help at all. It is difficult to distinguish which symptoms in women are caused by lower levels of oestrogen, and which are just the effects of ageing.

Physical causes

In women, physical effects of the menopause that can affect the enjoyment of sexual intercourse are that the breasts and clitoris become less responsive to stimulation, and muscle contractions during orgasm become weaker. Also, some women develop painful contractions of the womb during orgasm, which can be equally off-putting. Men of around this age may be starting to find that an erection takes longer to achieve, and is harder to maintain, so physical factors in both partners can contribute to a failing sexual relationship.

Psychological causes

Anxiety is a big passion-killer, and the middle years can produce a whole range of anxieties – problems with your children, worries about your ageing parents, suspicions that your husband might be interested in another woman, or even that he might have a heart attack during love-making.

Any one of these would be enough to make you feel like saying, 'Not tonight, dear, I've got a headache'.

Depression can reduce both men's and women's levels of desire to absolute zero. If your depression is directly related to the fall in your level of oestrogen, then there is a good chance that HRT can make you feel your old self again. It's therefore very important, if you see your GP about feeling depressed, that you also tell him about your other menopausal symptoms, so that he can link the depression to the menopause. If you don't, he may simply prescribe anti-depressants, and if your problem is caused by a drop in oestrogen, then anti-depressants will do nothing at all to tackle the underlying problem, and may just make you feel very much worse.

Stress and tension are common during the middle years, and can be made worse if you and your husband find it hard to communicate with each other. Women have conflicting roles at this time. Perhaps you are trying to rec-oncile the problems of being, simultaneously, a wife, a mother, a grandmother, a daughter and perhaps even a mistress. Each role makes quite different demands on you. Your mother may have perfected the art of 'putting you down', and making you feel still a child. Your grandchil-dren, on the other hand, probably think you are very, very old!

Medical causes

It is quite usual for people with various medical problems to find their interest in sex drops. This could be due to a whole range of physical disabilities, or to medical conditions they suffer from, or to medication that they take.

People, particularly men, who have had one heart attack, often have a natural fear that sexual intercourse may trigger another, and this is something your doctor (or the British Heart Foundation, see page 125) can advise you about.

Gynaecological or urinary problems can make women reluctant to have sexual intercourse, and some operations can cause changes to a woman's vagina or a man's penis so that sex becomes difficult or impossible. Many drugs reduce sexual desire, so if you have noticed your interest in sex dropping soon after starting a different course of medicine, ask your doctor about this, and he may feel it is possible to change the prescription.

Social causes

One of the social factors that contributes to sexual problems is alcohol; it affects a man's ability to achieve and maintain an erection, and a woman's ability to produce enough lubrication. Many older men and women drink much more than they did in their youth.

Another is the lack of a sexual partner due to death, divorce or separation, and the decreasing opportunities to find another as you get older. Most older women would be restrained by their upbringing from seeking a sexual partner other than within a fairly permanent relationship. One way in which many women choose to keep their sexual interest alive is by masturbation. Some religions do still prohibit it, but contrary to traditional church and public-school thinking, masturbation does not make you either blind or mad, nor is it unnatural, degrading or a form of 'beastliness'. It certainly isn't something you should feel guilty about. During the course of their lives, most people masturbate; and although men do it more than women, and younger people more than older people, there is nothing abnormal or unnatural about masturbation at any age. Many women feel it is no more or less satisfying than having sex with a partner, just different. In fact, for women who are unable for any reason to have sexual relations now but who feel they might want to in the future, it is a good way of keeping their 'sexual apparatus' functioning well, by maintaining their sexual responsiveness, by producing regular vaginal lubrication with mucus, and by keeping the necessary muscles in good working order. Sexual pleasure is closely linked with how well your vagina is working – a case of 'use it or lose it'; so if you feel that masturbation is right for you, then don't stifle this natural urge.

How HRT can help

It is not unusual for women to feel an increased sex drive after the menopause. This is often because they no longer have an underlying worry about becoming pregnant, although the majority of women now have available much more effective contraception than their mothers and grand-mothers did. However, if your sex drive has taken a plunge in your menopausal years, then HRT may help. Sometimes oestrogen alone is enough, but if loss of sex drive is coupled with a severe loss of self-confidence, your doctor may suggest you try the implant form of HRT as the male hormone, testosterone, can be incorporated into it, which may help these particular problems.

The male view

While on the subject of testosterone, how are things for your husband or partner at this time? As men don't menstruate, they can't technically be said to have a menopause, but from about their mid-forties, the level of testosterone in a man starts to fall gradually. Unlike women's oestrogen, it doesn't drop dramatically in their middle years, and sperm and testosterone production continue in men indefinitely, albeit at reducing levels. This is why men can father children right into old age. It seems rather unfair, doesn't it, that if a man in his fifties leaves his wife to have a new relationship with a younger woman, he can start a second family; the wife in her fifties can start a new relationship with a younger or an older man, but there will be no children of that union.

Falling levels of testosterone can decrease a man's sexual desire, and this in itself may make him irritable and depressed. He may find he can't get an erection so quickly, or sustain it for so long, and his wife may interpret this as a loss of interest in her, or that she is no longer attractive to him. If his falling hormone levels reduce his ability to perform as well sexually as he used to, his self-esteem may suffer. Add to this the fact that he may now be putting on weight, losing his youthful vitality, stuck in his job just for the pension, and feeling that it is now too late to make changes, and he may well try to revive his flagging self-esteem by playing energetic games of squash, starting a body-building course, or having an affair with a younger woman.

Perhaps he doesn't realise that both he and his wife are suffering from falling levels of their sex hormones, and it is having much the same effect on both of them. If his wife no longer wants sexual intercourse because a dry vagina makes it painful, and if her body no longer responds to the stimulation they have both enjoyed in the past, then he might feel rejected by her. It doesn't mean she doesn't love him, just that her hormones are affecting the way she feels, just as his are affecting him. Impotence in middle-aged men often happens as their wives reach the menopause: her lack of arousal and his inability to sustain an erection may make him feel frustrated, inadequate and even angry, and he needs her love and consideration at this time just as much as she needs his.

Many a wife gets into bed at night with her beer-bellied husband who is unshaven, slightly drunk, smelling of stale cigarettes, and who then complains that his wife 'doesn't want sex any more'. Well, can you blame her? The typical Englishman shaves when he gets out of bed in the morning, not when he gets into bed at night – what does that say about his efforts to make himself attractive to his wife?

Once you and your partner get out of the habit of sharing sex together, you may find it very difficult to start again. If you find sexual arousal is taking longer, try allowing yourself more time; or perhaps it might be more satisfying to have sex in the morning or afternoon when you are not tired or have not had too much food or drink to dull the senses. Try sharing a warm bath with pleasant additives, or using sensual massage on each other.

When he finds an erection difficult to sustain, and she has a less well lubricated vagina, it's all too easy to give up a form of sharing that is unlike any other. But don't feel you have to go along with society's view that 'people don't do it when they get older'. They can and they do, and if that's what feels right for you, so can you.

Chapter 6

Avoiding osteoporosis

‘Osteoporosis and its consequences may be regarded as one of the most serious long-term consequences of the human menopause.’ from *Focus – The Menopause*, International Monograph Series, 1990.

‘We are all aware of the undoubted benefits of HRT in preventing bone loss.’ letter in *British Medical Journal*, 1990.

It is possible that you have read this far through the book without having a very clear idea of what osteoporosis is. You probably know that it is something to do with bones, and from your reading of previous chapters that hormone replacement therapy seems to help prevent it. But what exactly is it? How serious is it? How likely are you to get it? And what can you do to prevent or treat it?

What is osteoporosis?

Osteoporosis is not life-threatening, in the sense that it will not kill you directly, but at its worst it can reduce your quality of life almost to zero, and can be an indirect cause of death. It is a much under-estimated disease, both in the number of women (and men) who suffer from it, and in the effect it has on their lives.

Perhaps you (or your mother) fell, landed on an out-stretched hand, and sustained a Colles' fracture of the wrist. That is almost certainly due to osteoporosis, especially if it happened some years after the menopause. Perhaps your mother or grandmother had a stoop known as a 'Dowager's Hump', and lost several inches in height. That is osteoporosis. Almost certainly you know an elderly person who has had a fractured hip. That, too, is osteoporosis.

By the age of 60, one woman in four will have had one or more fractures due to osteoporosis, and thousands in their fifties already have fractures of the spinal vertebrae. By the age of 80, half of all women will have had a fracture due to osteoporosis. And it is a depressing fact that of those who sustained a fractured hip, about one-quarter will have died within a year, and 50 per cent will no longer be able to live independently on their own.

In 1822, an eminent doctor called Sir Astley Cooper wrote: 'Our wards are seldom without an example of fracture of the upper part of the thigh bone.' He was talking about what nowadays we call a broken hip. Today, patients with broken hips occupy 20 per cent of all orthopaedic beds in the UK, and the incidence of osteoporosis is growing faster than the number of elderly people in the population.

Although doctors are concerned about the number of fractured hips because of the enormous cost to the NHS, the form of osteoporosis that causes the greatest pain, deformity and reduced quality of life is fracture of the vertebrae of the spine, a condition that usually starts when a woman is in her fifties or sixties, though in women who had a very early menopause, the first fracture may occur in her forties or even earlier. As each vertebra fractures (sometimes painlessly, sometimes causing excruciating pain), the spine can become bent, and the digestive organs, lungs and bladder become compressed, causing digestive, breathing and continence problems, and also a mortality level 15 per cent higher than without the fractures. As the spine becomes more curved, the abdomen protrudes, and clothes hang so badly it is difficult to look really good in anything. It is not unusual to lose up to 6 inches or more in height. For many women with severe osteoporosis, the feeling is, 'I hate what I have become.'

Obviously, osteoporosis is something you really do not want to get.

What causes osteoporosis?

As a simple definition, osteoporosis is a condition in which bone becomes so fragile and brittle that it breaks comparatively easily. Bone is a living, changing thing, containing two main types of cells called, confusingly, 'osteoclasts' and 'osteoblasts'. All through our lives, the osteoclasts wear away microscopic craters in the bone, and then the osteoblasts fill these craters with newly formed bone, exactly matching the space dissolved away by the osteoclasts. That way, bone is constantly renewed – a sort of repair-and-maintenance system. Oestrogen is thought to reduce the rate at which osteoclasts dissolve bone, and to increase the rate at which osteoblasts build it up. Once oestrogen levels fall, the osteoclasts dissolve the tiny craters at a faster rate than before, while the osteoblasts don't replace the bone so efficiently. Eventually, the bone becomes less dense and strong, and more liable to fracture.

Bone is built up during childhood and teenage years, and reaches a peak content (called 'peak bone mass') in the early twenties. For the next 15 years or so, the bones thicken and strengthen, but then from about the age of 35 onwards, bone mass starts to fall gradually. In a man it continues in this gradual fall for the rest of his life, and a man of 90 can expect to have lost about 25 per cent of his total quantity of bone. In women, however, bone density drops dramatically in the years immediately after the menopause – about 3–5 per cent every year in the vertebrae of women who have had a natural menopause, and as high as 7–9 per cent in the vertebrae of women who have had an early oophorectomy. (The hip joint loses bone density at a slightly lower rate.) To lose bone at about 3 per cent a year may not seem much, but if you get a calculator, start with 100 (to represent the amount of bone you have at the menopause), then subtract 3 per cent from that figure, then 3 per cent again from the next figure, you will find that after doing this seven times you get a figure of 80. In other words, after losing 3 per cent of your bone every year for seven years, you are left with just 80 per cent of what you had at the start of the menopause – and you are probably still only in your fifties. Many women lose bone mass at a faster rate than 3 per cent, and sometimes for as long as 15 or 20 years; it is not unusual for them to end up having lost one-third or even half of their bone mass by about the age of 70. No wonder fractures occur!

Bones are not solid things, like an iron bar, as this would make them very heavy. Each bone contains an outer shell of 'cortical' bone, which is strong, compact and dense, and an inner area of 'trabecular' bone, which is brittle and fragile. The bones that are most vulnerable to fracture in osteoporosis are those that have a higher proportion of trabecular bone, such as the hip joints and the vertebrae of the spine.

Trabecular bone is made up of tiny vertical pillars, joined together with horizontal cross-ties, giving it strength with the minimum of weight. In osteoporosis, as the osteoclasts wear away bone faster than the osteoblasts can build it up again, these pillars and cross-ties lose their connections with each other, and the bone therefore loses its strength. Eventually, it becomes so fragile that it can fracture while you are doing such everyday things as lifting a casserole out of the oven, opening a stuck window, putting shopping bags into the boot of the car, doing up the back zip of a dress, or even coughing, laughing or sneezing.

The main component of bone is calcium, which is held in a soft substance called collagen; as collagen levels fall, so do the levels of the calcium held within it. Oestrogen helps the body to absorb calcium effectively, making it available to the osteoblasts, and as oestrogen levels fall after the menopause, so calcium is stored less effectively. Much of it is just excreted in the urine instead of being used to build bone.

As oestrogen is needed to get the 'bone building' balance right, and as it also helps the body to absorb calcium and preserve collagen, you can see why oestrogen therapy is so effective in preventing osteoporosis. It can't rebuild damaged bone, but it can help prevent further bone loss. It has been said of HRT that it 'stops osteoporosis in its tracks', because oestrogen therapy at any stage after the menopause halts bone loss.

Can anyone get osteoporosis?

Yes, in the sense that we *all* lose bone from about the age of 35 or so. As men start with much bigger, stronger bones than women, they are much less likely to get it, and so are women who have big bones. You are most at risk of developing osteoporosis if:

- you had a menopause (surgical or natural) before about the age of 40 or 45
- you have a medical condition that requires you to take cortico-steroids in high doses for several years
- you have had a Colles' fracture of the wrist after the menopause, following a comparatively minor fall
- you have suffered from anorexia nervosa or bulimia
- you had amenorrhoea (absence of periods) for several years during your normal reproductive years

Other factors which increase your chance of getting osteoporosis are if:

- you are white or Asian
- you are small-boned, light in weight, and slender in build
- your mother, grandmothers or aunts had it
- you finished the menopause 10 or more years ago
- throughout most of your life you have eaten a diet low in calcium

However, people who don't fall into any of these categories can get osteoporosis.

These are mostly things you can't do anything about. There are some things you *can* do something about which contribute to osteoporosis:

- smoking (which lowers the natural level of oestrogen, and brings on the menopause up to five years earlier than it would otherwise have started)
- drinking large quantities of alcohol (which reduces the absorption of calcium from the digestive system, and slows down the activity of bone-forming osteoblasts)
- taking little or no weight-bearing exercise (bones get stronger when they are well used, and weaken when they are seldom used)
- dieting so severely that your periods (and thus your oestrogen production) stop
- continuing to have a diet low in calcium

When should HRT be taken to prevent osteoporosis?

The important word here is 'prevent'. At the moment there is no treatment that will significantly replace bone that has been lost. Once bone is lost through osteoporosis, it is, for all practical purposes, lost forever. Spinal vertebrae that become deformed through osteoporosis remain deformed forever. If you are at risk of developing a condition which is virtually irreversible, prevention becomes very important.

There is considerable evidence to show that starting oestrogen therapy within two years of the menopause, and staying on it for at least five years, can reduce your risk of getting a fracture of the hip or of a vertebra by 50 per cent. If you have had an early menopause you will have more years without oestrogen ahead of you, so you will need to stay on it for longer, probably until 65 or 70. Obviously HRT is more effective if started early and before you have lost much of your bone mass, but it really is never too late to start. In the United States, women sometimes go on it for the first time after a fractured hip in their nineties! Even in quite elderly women, HRT can slow bone loss.

What happens when you stop taking HRT?

When you are no longer taking oestrogen, the osteoclasts start dissolving bone away faster than the osteoblasts can replace it, and calcium in your diet is used less effectively. Therefore, you will start to lose bone again at about the same rate you would have lost it if you were not taking HRT. However, even five years on HRT will 'buy' you five years' delay in developing osteoporosis, which may make all the difference to getting a fractured hip or a bent spine. In an older person, this difference between getting or not getting a fracture can mean the difference between life and death.

What effect does progestogen have on osteoporosis?

One advantage of progestogen is that it does not appear to counteract the beneficial effects of oestrogen in building bone. It may even give some increase in bone density. So if you are unable to take oestrogen because of a medical condition, and you are worried about osteoporosis, progestogen on its own may help you.

How can you tell if you have osteoporosis?

Imagine you are quietly going about your normal life, when suddenly you trip and fall. You stretch out a hand to save yourself, and the next thing you know you have fractured your wrist. Unfortunately, most Accident and Emergency doctors are so busy that they just don't have time to explain that your Colles' fracture is probably caused by osteoporosis, even less to explain what you might do about it. An

X-ray will have shown up the fracture, but osteoporosis does not show up on an ordinary X-ray until one-quarter or more of the bone density has been lost, so if you have lost less than that so far the chances are that no one will notice that the cause of your fracture was osteoporosis, let alone tell you about it, and what you can do to stop it getting worse. A Colles' fracture should be seen as a warning sign about the state of your bones, while still giving you time to do something about it.

Sudden or severe backache in the years after the menopause can have many causes, and it may not occur to your doctor that osteoporosis could be the cause in your case. He may arrange an X-ray (which doesn't show any-thing wrong), possibly physiotherapy, probably painkillers, but eventually you get the message that you will 'just have to learn to live with it'.

It needn't be like that. Dual energy X-ray absorptiome-ter machines, known as DEXA (or DXA) for short, are the best way to screen bones for osteoporosis, and are now becoming available all over the country, both on the NHS and privately. DEXA scanning is quite painless, and involves no undressing or embarrassment. DEXA machines scan your hip and spine, and produce a reading of your bone density, which will give a good idea of whether or not you have got osteoporosis, how severe it is, and what your chances are of getting a fracture; the lower your bone den-sity, the more likely you are to sustain a fracture. Bone mineral density at the time of the menopause is the best predictor of osteoporosis, so in an ideal world, all women who are at risk of developing this disease would have a DEXA bone scan when they reached the menopause, and if their bone density was lower than it should be they would be advised on ways of reducing their chances of get-ting a fracture, including information on HRT. Until this happy day comes, don't ignore any back pain you get, or a Colles' fracture of the wrist, or loss of height – ask your doctor about osteoporosis.

You may see advertisements offering private screening for osteoporosis, and if this is on a DEXA bone scanner and will scan your hip and vertebrae, the reading will give your doctor a clear idea of your bone density and therefore of how likely you are to develop osteoporosis. Some companies are jumping on the osteoporosis bandwagon and offering screening that is less reliable; if you are in any doubt, ask your doctor. As a general rule, the only way to tell what the bone density is in your hip is to scan the hip, and the same with the vertebrae; scanning other parts of the body (such as the heel and wrist) does not give a truly accurate impression of your bone density in the important hip and spine areas. However, such a scan will show if your bone density is very low or very high; it's those people in the middle who will need more precise measurement.

Scanning poses a difficult dilemma for the National Health Service. To scan all post-menopausal women would be prohibitively expensive, and large-scale trials have shown that it is not cost-effective to do this. To scan all women who are at risk of developing osteoporosis is still expensive, but if it can reduce the number of osteoporotic fractures (which currently cost the NHS over £600 million a year) by identifying women who have a low bone density and offering them treatment, such as HRT, to reduce their chance of having a hip fracture, then considerable savings can be made. On the other hand, if millions of women take HRT for many years, that, too, is very expensive.

If I am unable or unwilling to take HRT, what else can be done about osteoporosis?

The most effective way of reducing your chances of an osteoporotic fracture are to build up your bone mass during your youth by taking plenty of exercise (which strengthens bones), by eating a diet high in calcium, by avoiding drastic dieting and by not smoking. This ensures that you reach the menopause with your bones as strong as your basic genetic make-up allows.

From the menopause onwards you need to continue with exercise, and with calcium in your diet. Many women worry about putting on weight at this time, so they cut down on the dairy products that contain calcium to protect their bones, which is a pity. If you take very little calcium in your diet, calcium supplements may be helpful (see Chapter 9). Bones also need a small amount of vitamin D, and for most people, the best way to take in vitamin D is to expose your skin to sunlight: about 30 minutes a day in winter and summer is ideal, long enough for the vitamin to be produced in the skin, not long enough to run the risk of skin cancer. Large doses of vitamin D (as are found in some tablets, for example) can actually be harmful to bones.

If you have osteoporosis of the spine, your doctor will be able to tell you about a new treatment called etidronate, marketed by Norwich Eaton under the brand name of Didronel PMO. This is a non-hormonal treatment, so it is suitable for many women who cannot take HRT. It has the advantage that, taken regularly, it can lead to a small build-up of bone that has been lost. It is taken on a cyclical basis – 14 days of etidronate followed by 76 days of calcium supplements. This cycle is then repeated over and over for three years or more. Didronel PMO appears to have few side-effects (mainly minor stomach upsets) but, being non-hormonal, it does not give any improvement of menopausal symptoms. It is only available on prescription, is particularly suitable for older women, although there is no upper or lower recommended age, and is intended as a treatment for osteoporosis of the spine, not of the hip. Didronel PMO is also likely to be helpful to men who suffer from osteoporosis.

Whether or not you decide to take hormone replacement therapy to prevent or delay osteoporosis, is a decision you will want to make after thinking about it carefully. Although it is never too late to start, for it to be most effective you should take it for at least five years, preferably starting within two or three years of the menopause. If you are at a high risk of developing osteoporosis, a much longer period may be necessary for you, and you will need to balance the slightly increased risk of developing breast cancer (if you take it for 10 or 15 years or more) against the risk of developing a condition that can cause considerable pain and deformity.

For decades, women suffered in silence from osteoporosis, while their doctors regarded it as just one of the consequences of old age – inevitable, unpreventable, untreatable and boring. It has recently been described as 'a preventable disease that is not being prevented, a treatable disease that is not being treated'. Even in 1990, out of the 2 million women in the UK who suffer from this condition, only 76,000 received any treatment at all, and 90 per cent of those received only calcium and painkillers. Only a tiny minority received HRT.

Things are changing at last, however. More and more women have heard of osteoporosis, and know what it is. Doctors have a clearer idea of how to diagnose and treat it. It is becoming a high-profile disease, the subject of hundreds of research projects in the UK alone. That this is happening is due almost entirely to the work of the National Osteoporosis Society (see page 126). Founded in 1986, it now has over 14,000 members, with local groups in most parts of the country. The Society aims to keep osteoporosis very much in the public eye, to raise money for research, to make sure government ministers and the Department of Health are constantly aware of the enormous amount of work that still needs to be done in research, bone scanning, treatment, prevention campaigns, etc. The National Osteoporosis Society has regular programmes to up-date doctors about osteoporosis so that they can help their patients more. It runs information campaigns on osteoporosis in pregnancy, osteoporosis in men, the importance of screening and of HRT, and, very importantly, to make sure that all sufferers receive treatment. If you want to know where you can get your bone density measured; if there is a consultant special-ising in osteoporosis in your area; how to cope with living with the disease; what to do about exercise, diet, calcium supplements, etc; if you wish your doctor knew more about osteoporosis and how to help you; if you want to know more about the role of HRT in the prevention and treat-ment of osteoporosis; if you would like to get together with other local sufferers; or if you just want someone to reach out a sympathetic hand . . . then join the National Osteo-porosis Society. They have members in their twenties and thirties through to their eighties and nineties. Whether you have osteoporosis now, or are worried you may get it one day in the future, why not give your support to the organi-sation that is working to help everyone with this condition.

(For further reading on osteoporosis, a book I wrote in 1990 goes into more detail. It's called *Everything You Need To Know About Osteoporosis*, and is published by Sheldon Press.)

Chapter 7

It isn't all roses – the disadvantages and contraindications of HRT

‘Few therapies in the medical field have generated such controversy as that of hormone replacement.’ from *Medical Clinics of North America*, 1987.

One day, possibly, medicine will come up with a treatment that is 100 per cent effective, 100 per cent safe, and totally without side-effects in anybody. But don't hold your breath!

Hormone replacement has many advantages, particularly in improving the quality of life for women at, or beyond, the menopause. With the exception of heart attack or stroke, the symptoms of low oestrogen are not life-threatening; women are not going to die from hot flushes, tiredness, loss of continence, or even directly from osteoporosis. But all these things greatly reduce their self-image, self-esteem and general enjoyment of life. So any treatment that can improve these conditions would seem to be well worth considering.

HRT, like every treatment for every condition currently available on the traditional medical market, has its drawbacks. But it's the best we've got at the moment, and millions of women derive great benefit from it: their hot flushes disappear, sex becomes enjoyable again, and their chance of getting osteoporosis or heart disease is greatly reduced. Many also notice an improvement in the quality of their skin and hair, in reduced muscle and joint pains, in increased energy and vitality and in their sense of well-being.

Why, then, are only 9 per cent of menopausal and post-menopausal women in the UK taking HRT at any one time, and why do most give up after just a few months?

> ❝I felt quite bloated, and had headaches and breast tenderness.❞

> ❝After three months I just couldn't cope with having periods again.❞

> ❝HRT certainly helped my hot flushes, but I gave up after putting on weight.❞

> ❝It made me feel irritable and depressed.❞

> ❝I am afraid of breast cancer.❞

> ❝The patch made my skin red and itchy, so I changed to tablets, but they caused heart palpitations.❞

> ❝Fluid retention and leg cramps made me feel really uncomfortable.❞

> ❝My doctor doesn't believe in it.❞

> ❝I just don't think it's natural.❞

The main reasons why women don't even start taking HRT are the feeling that it is 'going against nature', together with a lack of knowledge of how it works and why replacing oestrogen after the menopause can be such a good thing.

> ❝I think HRT is interfering with nature, and I can't imagine that I would ever want to use it. It seems all wrong to me.❞

The two commonest reasons why women who are already on HRT give it up are a dislike of monthly bleeds, especially among those well past the menopause, and the fear of breast cancer, which is shared by doctors and patients alike. Other real turn-offs are the need to take a pill every day (or change a patch every few days), the cost of prescriptions for the under-sixties, a slight weight gain and nausea, a return to pre-menstrual tension (if you take progestogen), and the need for regular gynaecological check-ups. This chapter looks at these, and also at who may be advised not to take it at all for medical reasons.

In addition to those who give up HRT for all the above reasons, there are those who do so because it doesn't relieve their symptoms. Unfortunately, most women who give up because of side-effects have only ever tried one form of HRT. But as you will realise by now, if you get either no relief, or undesirable side-effects, the many combinations of oestrogen and progestogen on the market should mean that you can eventually find one that is right for you. If you are to find the right one, you may have to persevere for several months, trying out different preparations, and this will obviously mean several return visits to the doctor. A survey of women conducted in 1992 by The Amarant Trust (see page 125) found that women who had received only brief and inadequate information on HRT when they were first prescribed it, were very much more likely to give up after only a few months than women whose doctors had taken the time and trouble to explain about the menopause, about how HRT works, and to give them a realistic idea of possible side-effects. Don't be afraid of being thought a member of The Awkward Squad: it's your body, and oestrogen replacement could make all the difference to your present well-being and future health.

Side-effects of hormone replacement therapy

The commonest side-effects are:

- feelings of nausea
- breast tenderness

- feeling bloated before a period
- slight weight-gain
- disturbances of the digestive system
- leg cramps
- headaches
- feelings of pre-menstrual tension and other complaints caused by taking progestogen

Although this may seem a daunting list, most of these problems are quite short-lived for the majority of women on HRT.

Feelings of nausea

These usually wear off quite quickly, and are much less of a problem with the patch and implant than with tablets.

Breast tenderness

This, too, usually wears off after the first week or two. If it is troublesome, it may be relieved by starting with a low dose of oestrogen and building up once your body has become used to having the hormone again.

Feeling bloated

This is caused by fluid retention, and may include swollen ankles. Talk to your doctor about it; he may prescribe 'water tablets', or the symptoms may subside by themselves.

Weight gain

This is usually short-lived. A small minority gain five pounds or more, but even those who put on weight at the start of HRT usually end up only about one pound heavier than when they started. Allow yourself two or three months for your body to adjust before worrying about any extra weight – you'll probably lose it anyway, although the progestogen stage of the cycle may cause a weight gain of two or three pounds, like it did before the menopause, and this is lost again when the course of progestogen finishes. As we get older, we all start to burn calories more slowly than we did in our youth, so if you are eating the same amount of food as you did several years ago you will end up putting on weight unless you can take more exercise to burn it up. A thickening of the waist is not quite the same as weight gain, and is due to getting older, not to HRT. Before the menopause, a woman produces mainly female hormones, but also a small amount of male hormones too; the oestrogen causes the typical female shape of large breasts and hips and a small waist. But when oestrogen falls, the male hormones start to predominate, so the older woman tends to have a thicker waist, smaller breasts and a deeper voice.

Many of those who gain more weight are smokers who have been advised to give up smoking while they are on HRT – so they eat instead! Others lose weight on HRT. These are often women who were distressed and unhappy because of menopausal symptoms and who used to eat to 'comfort' themselves. Once on HRT they feel happier in themselves, so don't feel the need to eat so much.

Disturbances of the digestive system (known as gastro-intestinal disturbances)

These are more common with oral HRT than with other types. If you take the oral form, these symptoms are often relieved by taking the tablet with food, or at bedtime; if this doesn't help, a non-oral route like the patch or implant may solve the problem.

Leg cramps

Cramp, especially in the calves, sometimes occurs in the first few months of taking HRT. It may be worse at night, and usually disappears before long. If you regularly get cramp in one leg only, mention it to your GP, who will want to check that you are not at risk of developing a thrombosis.

Headaches

These are usually short-lived, too. If you developed migraine at the time of the menopause, HRT may relieve it; if the HRT causes headaches, they should pass, but if they don't your doctor may suggest changing the dosage or type.

PMT and other symptoms of progestogen

These have been covered in Chapter 3. Again, the patch form of progestogen may see the end of many of these troublesome complaints, so should the newer progestogens when they become available.

Other disadvantages of taking HRT

For women who still have a uterus, a return to monthly bleeds is usually a complete turn-off. And the further past the menopause they are, the more of a turn-off it seems. Not many 60- and 70-year-olds would willingly go back to all that again. But the interesting thing is that they do, especially if they have, or are at risk of, osteoporosis.

As with most medical treatments, if the benefits of the treatment substantially outweigh the disadvantages, then people will continue with it. At present, the great majority of women who stay on HRT for any length of time are those who have had a hysterectomy; the highest drop-out rate is among those who need to take progestogen and who therefore have 'periods' and other side-effects.

Women who have just reached the menopause are usually delighted to see an end to their periods in sight, until the hot flushes come along. Then having a monthly bleed seems somehow less troublesome than coping with the flushes. For those, however, who are only mildly troubled with them, the thought of continuing with periods is probably out of proportion to the small discomfort of the flushes. The decision will be yours.

Many women over 60 seem willing to accept a return to periods once they realise they are likely to be regular, predictable and usually light; in fact they eventually become little more than just 'spotting'. Perhaps part of the older woman's aversion to periods is her memory of bulky sanitary towels, belts, even plastic 'sanitary pants'. Nowadays, every older woman has at least heard of tampons, even if she never quite got round to using them, and advertisements for slim-line sanitary towels that stick on to pants appear regularly on television. You can forget the bulk, the belt, the plastic pants. With tampons and slim pads you would hardly know you had a period. Honestly! Even buying them in shops is not the awful embarrassment it used to be — just pick them off the shelf in the chemist or supermarket and they are discreetly wrapped at the till.

How happily you return to periods will depend on your perception of the trade-off between symptoms and periods, and on your doctor's attitude to HRT. If he is fairly negative, then he will probably portray periods in a negative light; if he is enthusiastic, his enthusiasm may make you feel altogether better about it.

Eventually, with luck, 'no-bleed HRT' will be what we all get offered. So far, just one type — Livial — is available (as described on page 50), but other pharmaceutical companies will bring out their own brands over the next few years. There is no doubt that this form of HRT will greatly increase the proportion of women who (a) even consider starting hormone replacement, and (b) remain on it for a long time.

A comparatively minor disadvantage of being on HRT is the need for regular gynaecological check-ups. Doctors, like policemen, get younger every day, and most older women don't like the idea of being given a breast and vaginal check-up by a younger male doctor. Yes, he has certainly seen it all before, and yes, he regards the genital area with the same disinterest with which he regards noses and ears, but even so the average older woman (and younger woman too) can find these check-ups embarrassing.

It is worth making two points here: Firstly, you may not need to see a young male doctor. Most GP practices nowadays have at least one woman doctor, so you might prefer to see her. Or perhaps the practice has a Menopause Nurse who specialises in all aspects of the menopause and does these check-ups every day. Failing that, you could go to your local Well Woman Clinic, where all the staff are women, and to which you don't need to be referred by your doctor. Secondly, the regular check-up really is to your advantage. It will probably include a cervical smear (to detect any possible cancer of the cervix), a breast check (to detect any possible breast cancer or other abnormality), and a check on your weight, blood pressure and, possibly, cholesterol. Conditions that might have developed unnoticed will be picked up early; these regular check-ups really could save your life.

Can anyone take hormone replacement therapy?

No. If you have certain medical conditions (as detailed on pages 88–90), your doctor may decide that HRT would not be a particularly good idea. If you have certain other conditions (see opposite), he may refuse to prescribe it for you at all. Whether you can (or should) take HRT depends on your doctor's assessment of the risks involved, and whether you have 'relative contraindications' or 'absolute contraindications'.

'Risk' means the likelihood of a condition developing as a direct result of a particular treatment. In the case of HRT, this usually refers to the risk of cancer, specifically breast cancer.

'Contraindication' means that a condition you already have may get worse if you take the treatment. Circumstances in which HRT should not be prescribed (except in very particular cases) are 'absolute contraindications'; 'relative contraindications' refer to situations in which it can usually be prescribed, but which need careful assessment and monitoring, and only certain types may be advisable (such as the patch, for example, in order to avoid the liver and digestive system).

The generally accepted **absolute contraindications**, that is circumstances in which HRT should never usually be prescribed, are:

- cancer of the endometrium (lining of the womb)
- breast cancer
- if you are pregnant, or think that you might be
- abnormal vaginal bleeding which has not been investigated and the cause diagnosed
- severe liver disease where the liver is not functioning normally

In addition to these, most doctors would be very reluctant to prescribe HRT if you have or have had:

- a stroke
- a recent heart attack
- a recent thrombosis
- disease of the pancreas
- disease of the gallbladder
- otosclerosis (a rare form of progressive irreversible deafness)

There are, however, some women who suffer from these conditions yet still take HRT. Just occasionally, a doctor will feel that a particular woman is suffering so severely from menopausal symptoms that her whole quality of life is being reduced almost to zero; she may even feel suicidal. In these cases, a doctor may decide, having explained the risks to her, that a low dosage of HRT may be the most suitable treatment. She would obviously need to understand that, for example, a cancerous tumour or a liver condition may get worse, but she does at least have the right to choose, and she will make the decision having been given all the information. For many people, quality of life is more important than quantity, and women who feel this may decide to take

HRT knowing that it may make an existing condition worse, and may even shorten their life. That is their decision. Others will decide that they will not risk making things worse, so they put up with severe menopausal symptoms as the lesser of two evils.

There is a long list of **relative contraindications** to HRT, that is those conditions in which you and your doctor will need to consider the balance between the risks and the benefits:

● **Angina, or if you have a family history of heart disease**, was previously thought to be an absolute contraindication, but with research now showing that HRT can offer positive protection against heart disease, medical opinion is changing about this. Your doctor will be able to advise you according to your particular condition, and may suggest a non-oral type, such as the patch or implant.

● The risk if you have had **deep vein thrombosis** depends on how any previous thrombosis occurred. If it first occurred after you had been bedridden for a long time because of illness or a major operation, such as a hip replacement, and especially if it happened long before the menopause, then your doctor may feel it is unlikely to happen again in normal circumstances, so HRT would probably be possible. However, if the thrombosis occurred for no apparent reason, then your doctor would probably want to investigate it, and may then decide against HRT in your case. If the thrombosis occurred while you used the contraceptive pill, he will probably advise against HRT.

● **Diabetics** can usually take HRT safely, but as it can affect the way carbohydrates are broken down in the body, very careful monitoring would be necessary, and the diabetes would need to be stabilised before a course of HRT was started.

● **Endometriosis** can lead to a difficult decision having to be made. If you had an oophorectomy, then you will probably have particularly troublesome hot flushes, and if you had the operation before about the age of 45 you will be at a much greater risk of developing osteoporosis, so HRT would seem an important treatment for you. However, the excess tissue that built up in endometriosis may get worse on HRT, even many years after the menopause, suggesting that you should not use this form of treatment. This is obviously something you should talk over with your doctor.

• If you have a **family history of cancer of the breast or uterus**, your doctor will want to consider what your chances are of developing either of these diseases if you take HRT. Once again, only you can decide by weighing the relative risks against the relative benefits. Benign breast disease needs careful monitoring, but HRT needn't always be ruled out.

• **Fibroids** tend to get worse in the presence of oestrogen, and may enlarge if you take HRT. But this doesn't usually cause extra problems and most women with fibroids who are on HRT find they just have heavier periods.

• The presence of **gallstones** means HRT has to be prescribed with caution, as it can lead to an increased risk of this condition becoming worse. A non-oral route, such as the patch or implant, avoids the digestive system, so may be acceptable. Oestrogen can make gallbladder disease worse.

• **High blood pressure** should be investigated before starting on HRT, but once it has been brought under control, your doctor will probably feel it is alright for you to be on HRT. High blood pressure is not in itself a contraindication.

• **Migraine** responds unpredictably to HRT, and your doctor may suggest you try it for a month or two to start with to see how it affects you. If you develop migraine for the first time during or after the menopause, then it may be

Some women find it returns during the days in each month when they are taking progestogen. Unfortunately, in these cases, changing to a different type of progestogen will probably not bring much improvement.

● Women who are **overweight** can usually take HRT, but very overweight women have a higher-than-average level of oestrogen, and increasing this level with HRT can increase the risk of breast cancer. However, these women, because of their higher oestrogen levels, tend to be less troubled by menopausal symptoms, and are at low risk of developing osteoporosis.

● There is no reason why **smokers** shouldn't take HRT, although some doctors advise them to give up smoking while they are on it. Smoking reduces oestrogen levels.

● **Varicose veins** are not usually connected with deep vein thrombosis, and if this is so for you then there is no reason why you can't take HRT unless they are acutely inflamed (phlebitis). Superficial inflammation of varicose veins is not a contraindication.

Between 10 and 20 per cent of post-menopausal women have significant contraindications to HRT, and the majority of them have menopausal symptoms that cause them long- or short-term embarrassment or distress. They need treatment to cope with the hot flushes, etc, and to increase their sense of wellbeing, yet many doctors aren't particularly helpful.

You and your doctor

Whether your doctor is enthusiastic about HRT or not is quite closely linked to how long ago he qualified. Most older doctors hardly studied even the menopause at medical school, and HRT not at all. A survey in Brighton, Sussex, showed that of doctors who qualified in the 1950s, none prescribed HRT in a given year, those who qualified in the

prescribed HRT in a given year, those who qualified in the 1960s were slightly more likely to, while those who qualified in the 1970s and 1980s were very likely to. So if your doctor is rather older than average and 'doesn't believe in HRT', you might find a younger doctor more helpful; and, no matter what his age, if you do not feel he is sympathetic to your problems, ask whether you could see another doctor in the practice, or a Menopause Nurse. If you get no luck there, a local Menopause Clinic or Well Woman Clinic will be able to give you the information you want, and do a medical check-up. Help, information, advice and treatment is also available from The Amarant Trust (address on page 125). The aim of the Trust is to promote a greater understanding of the menopause and HRT. They run an HRT helpline for general enquiries, can send you a list of NHS and private Menopause Clinics, run specialist courses for GPs and nurses, and have their own private Menopause Clinics in London and Cheshire, where patients can receive assessment, information and treatment.

Most women nowadays are much better informed on medical matters than their mothers or grandmothers were, and they expect to be given as much information as possible. You do not have to be putty in your doctor's hands; you don't have to take (or not take) medicine just because he says so; you have every right to full information and then to make your own mind up. Fortunately, the 'because-I-say-so, my dear, and-don't-ask-so-many-questions' type of doctor is becoming a dying breed, and GPs now expect their patients to want information about their condition and its treatment, including the options available and possible side-effects of different treatments. If you are unsure about anything, go along to your doctor with a list of questions written down on paper and then write his replies down, so you don't forget anything. By thinking about things in advance, you are less likely to come out of the surgery saying to yourself, 'Bother, I forgot to ask him about such-and-such.' You may prefer to take somebody into the consulting

and less intimidated, and you have the right to do this, and also to a second opinion.

As a result of the scares abut HRT in the 1970s, many doctors are uncertain how safe it is nowadays, and perhaps do not realise that cancer of the lining of the womb can virtually be ruled out for women starting HRT now as long as they take progestogen as well as oestrogen. They might also link safety concerns about the oral contraceptive with HRT, but as the dose is many times smaller, this is a largely unfounded fear. Although many doctors realise the benefits of long-term HRT for osteoporosis and heart attacks, they are also aware that there is an increased risk of breast cancer in women who take it long-term. It is interesting, though, that doctors involved in research projects with women who are taking HRT do seem to be enthusiastic about it; perhaps they feel it really does work, and, in most cases, has more advantages than disadvantages.

Finally, however well you are getting on with HRT, it is not a panacea for eternal good health, and any of us can develop serious diseases. There are some symptoms you should not ignore, whether or not you think they are connected with either the menopause or HRT:

- very heavy periods
- any bleeding or 'spotting' between periods
- any bleeding or 'spotting' after sexual intercourse
- any unexplained bleeding once the menopause has passed
- if you still haven't reached the menopause by about the age of 54
- pain or swelling in the abdomen
- 'indigestion'-type pain that persists for more than a day or two
- blood in the urine or stools

If you get any of these, see your doctor as soon as possible.

While a few GPs are still reluctant to take menopausal symptoms seriously ('No one yet died of the menopause, my dear'), many are both enthusiastic and helpful. An increas-

dear'), many are both enthusiastic and helpful. An increasing number have set up Menopause Clinics within their practices, employing specialist Menopause Nurses, from whom women can receive advice, information and screening. Newly pregnant women see their GPs, and all women approaching the menopause should be encouraged to do so as well, not necessarily to be given HRT, but to discuss the menopause, their symptoms, and any treatment that may be advisable. Women who are well informed about this time of change will feel better able to cope with it, and will not be a burden to themselves or to their doctors.

Chapter 8

Breast cancer – an understandable fear

‘I had a late menopause, and have been told that this might increase my chances of getting breast cancer, but my older sister has osteoporosis at 62, so I really don't know what to do.’

‘Breast cancer is what would really put me off HRT. In fact, I don't think I'd even consider taking it.’

‘My mother died of breast cancer, and my doctor said I shouldn't take HRT, but I've been feeling so low lately, so tired, and with awful hot flushes, that right now I think I'd honestly rather take the risk of dying slightly sooner from breast cancer. At least I'd enjoy the years until then.’

‘I really don't know what to think. I read about TV stars saying how young they feel on HRT, then I hear stories about breast cancer. Some of my friends have found it wonderful, others just didn't get on with it.’

‘One minute you read about how wonderful HRT is, and the next there's a breast cancer scare.’

‘Eleven out of 12 women don't get breast cancer.’

Breast cancer is one of the most controversial aspects of hormone replacement therapy. Fear of the disease is the main reason why women don't want to take it and why doctors are reluctant to prescribe it. No sooner had the risk of endometrial cancer in women taking HRT been largely overcome when up popped the spectre of breast cancer.

So what exactly are the risks? It is worth pointing out that breast cancer has been around since long before HRT, and that approximately one woman in 12 will develop it whether she is on HRT or not. So there is always this risk in the background.

There are various factors which increase your particular chances of developing breast cancer, whether you take HRT or not:

- If a very close relative, such as your mother or sister, developed breast cancer, although recent evidence suggests this may be less of a risk than was once thought.
- If you have 'benign' breast disease (your doctor would tell you if you have); this is not always a higher risk factor in itself, but as lumpy breasts make the detection of cancer more difficult, some doctors prefer their patients not to take HRT.
- If you finished your periods later than average, that is you had a late menopause (after about the age of 55).
- If you are very overweight.

None of these means that you *will* get breast cancer, just that your chances of getting it are higher than for women who don't fit into any of these categories.

From the last two in the list, you will see that there appears to be a link between oestrogen and breast cancer. In other words, women who have been producing oestrogen for longer than average have a higher than average risk of developing breast cancer. So, if these women take HRT for many years more, this risk will increase further, and this is something they should be aware of, so that they can make an informed decision. Even so, it is only a *risk*, not a certainty.

Conversely, you are at a lower than average risk of developing breast cancer if you had an early menopause (whether surgical or natural); the 'downside' for this group of women is that, because they produced oestrogen for a shorter than average time, they are at an increased risk of developing osteoporosis. It seems we really can't win!

Some breast cancer tumours depend on oestrogen to grow, and some don't. If your breast cancer developed before the menopause (that is, while you were still producing oestrogen), then HRT is a definite NO for you; but if it developed long afterwards, then in some cases HRT may be acceptable. This is a situation where you and your doctor will have to balance the risks against the benefits. It is obviously difficult to work out these risks and benefits. Most research identifies the risks to the population at large, whereas you want to know how it might affect *you* as an individual, regardless of how it might affect anybody else. Your doctor or specialist should be able to help you.

As a general guideline, the chances of developing breast cancer increase with the length of time you take HRT, and also the higher the dose of oestrogen. There appears to be no significant risk to women in the population at large who take it for less than five years, but the risk increases slightly between 5 and 10 years, and taking it for more than 15 years gives a higher risk still. (It is this long-term risk that has attracted media attention, though often the scare-mongering headlines are quite unjustified medically.) This can cause problems, because long-term oestrogen use is important for preventing osteoporosis, heart attack and stroke; and many women also feel so good on it that they would be very reluctant to give it up after just a few years.

Cancer is a very real fear for doctors and patients alike. Nobody wants to get it, but the risk needs to be put into perspective. Under the age of 50, deaths in women from breast cancer out-number deaths from coronary heart disease and stroke combined. However, after the age of 50, this ratio is reversed, and far more women die from a heart attack or stroke than from breast cancer. Oestrogen reduces by 50 per cent your chances of having a heart attack or stroke.

The risks of developing breast cancer as a direct result of taking HRT are small when set against the protection it confers against osteoporosis and arterial disease, although it is important to say here that if you take progestogen in the therapy, then some of the protection against heart attack may be reduced. Progestogen's effect on breast cancer is not clearly known; some researchers have concluded that it offers some protective effect, others that it may have a negative effect, and others still that it has no effect at all. More research is clearly needed here.

It is thought that oestrogens neither increase nor decrease the risk of cancer of the ovaries in post-menopausal women compared with those who do not take it; and oestrogen and progestogen appear to have no effect on the incidence of cancer of the cervix.

One important thing that has been noted is that, although there is a higher rate of breast cancer among women who take HRT than among those who don't, their *survival* rate is also higher. In other words, if you develop breast cancer and are on HRT, you have a better chance of surviving than if you develop breast cancer and are not on HRT. This is possibly because regular screening of women on HRT picks up any breast problems in the very early stages, when treatment is more likely to be effective. Some studies have also suggested that tumours linked to oestrogen therapy might be less virulent and invasive than other types of tumours, and that these particular tumours respond to treatment better than tumours not linked to oestrogen therapy.

A tremendous amount of research is being carried out into all aspects of HRT and the menopause. Hopefully, the time will come when doctors will know more clearly which particular sub-group of women would be more at risk of developing breast cancer if they took HRT, so that they can leave it well alone, and the rest can take it with confidence and safety.

Chapter 9
Managing the menopause without HRT

Hormone replacement therapy isn't right for every woman. Some can't take it because of medical conditions they either have or are at risk of having; some are completely turned off by the various side-effects; others don't want to take it because they believe it is unnatural, interfering with nature. Women who spent most of their reproductive years on the Pill may now want to have a break from all hormones; and many don't want to 'pop a pill every day' to prevent conditions they haven't got and may never have.

If you are in the lucky 20 per cent who sail through the menopause with hardly a symptom to complain about, you will probably not give HRT a second thought. Osteoporosis and heart attacks seem far away on life's distant horizon. However, if you feel you are at risk of developing either of these conditions, then HRT is a form of prevention you should think about – it is not just for treating hot flushes.

Of the remaining 80 per cent who get menopausal symptoms, only a very small proportion at present take HRT, although their number is now growing steadily as women understand more about it, and doctors feel more confident about prescribing it. Even so, many women are still unable or unwilling to receive hormone treatment, so what else is available for them at this time?

There are many and varied ways of coping with the different symptoms that afflict menopausal women. Some involve taking medication of different types, others involve making lifestyle changes. None of them is a true replacement for oestrogen, and it really is worth keeping this thought at the back of your mind, especially if you want to protect yourself from osteoporosis and coronary heart disease.

As we get older, we must work at being healthy. We can no longer abuse our bodies and expect to get away with it. The teenager or young woman who smokes, drinks and takes no exercise probably won't notice the effect for many years; for the older woman it is different – suddenly these habits affect her life *now*.

Smoking, coffee and alcohol all make vasomotor symptoms (hot flushes and night sweats) worse; alcohol and tobacco lower the oestrogen supply; alcohol also interferes with the body's effective use of calcium; taking no exercise increases the risk of getting osteoporosis and a heart attack. Isn't it unfair!

Hot flushes

Few treatments are as effective as oestrogen, but if oestrogen is not for you, then what else can you do? Firstly, try not to let your doctor prescribe tranquillisers, sedatives or anti-depressants; they don't relieve the hot flushes and night sweats, and they may make you feel much worse.

Controlling or preventing hot flushes is not easy, but some things make them worse, so:

- try to cut down on smoking, coffee and alcohol
- avoid hot spicy foods
- try to avoid stress
- ask your doctor if any tablets you are taking could be making the flushes worse
- wear cool, loose clothing made of natural fibres, especially in hot weather
- have a tepid shower whenever possible

- if you decide to stop HRT, do it as slowly as possible, and not during hot weather or times of stress

> ❝I stopped taking HRT to see if my ovaries would start working again without it, but they didn't, and the hot flushes came back. So I went back on the HRT and feel much better now. I am 52.❞

> ❝I bought some special "calcium tablets for women" from the health food shop for my flushes, but they didn't help at all.❞

The first of the two women quoted above doesn't understand that once ovaries have stopped 'working' after the menopause, they won't start up again. And the second has been misinformed about calcium tablets; they will help your bones, but not hot flushes.

Herbal remedies can sometimes help hot flushes; instead of just buying something over the counter at the chemist or health food shop, you might get a remedy that is more appropriate for you if you visit a medical herbalist or an aromatherapist. A homoeopath may also prescribe a suitable remedy (see address section of page 125). Bear in mind, though, that these remedies are not oestrogen, so will not prevent osteoporosis; however, many women find that alternative medicines can help other aspects of coping with the menopause.

Unlike vaginal and bladder problems, and osteoporosis, hot flushes will eventually pass for almost all women. They can be embarrassing and uncomfortable, and they may make you want to disappear into a hole in the ground, but they don't last forever. If you are lucky, they will be over in about two years or even less, and if these are your only symptoms you may well feel that HRT is not necessary for you; if you are one of the unlucky ones, the hot flushes may still be with you in 20 years, and HRT may be the only effective solution.

Dry skin

As you will have read in Chapter 1, skin blooms in the presence of oestrogen. Once you are producing little or no oestrogen, your skin gradually becomes drier and more wrinkled. To counteract this, many of the so-called moisturisers work by introducing moisture into the very top, thin layer of skin (the epidermis), so that it looks fuller and small wrinkles are eased out. But in the process of doing this, the epidermis stretches slightly to accommodate the moisturiser, so that when you stop using it, your skin starts to sag more than ever. The beautiful skin of a young woman (especially a pregnant young woman) is due to oestrogen acting on the thick underlying layer of skin (the dermis) and its collagen, which increases the moisture content of the skin. No amount of artificial moisturising in the thin top layer can produce this effect.

But you needn't start to look like an old hag the minute your periods stop! You just need to be aware of what makes your skin look older as time goes on, and time starts going on from about the age of 35!

Most damage to the skin is done by smoking and by excessive exposure to sunlight. Smoking reduces the blood supply to the skin cells by narrowing the tiny blood vessels; also the blood of a smoker carries less oxygen and more carbon monoxide than the blood of a non-smoker, so the cells of both the upper epidermis and the underlying dermis don't receive enough nourishment, and lose moisture. Yet another reason to stop smoking! In fact, if you look around you, you will notice that, on the whole, the natural 'un-moisturised' skin of older women tends to be less attractive in smokers than in non-smokers.

Too much sun on the skin can also damage the underlying layers, and make them less elastic. In excessive amounts it can also cause skin cancer. (As with smokers, you have probably noticed that the skin of a woman who has spent much time in a hot climate tends to be dryer and more wrinkled than the skin of a woman who has spent her summers in Britain.) But in small quantities, sunlight on the skin is the best possible way of taking in vitamin D, which plays a vital part in helping the body use calcium effectively to build good bones. So do get out into the sunshine for your bones, but don't overdo it.

Urinary problems

Embarrassing little dribbles can be a nightmare. The smell on your clothes and chairs, the tell-tale damp patches on your skirt or trousers, the awful wondering if anyone has noticed. You don't have to be Very Old to have continence problems; they can start when you are in your fifties, or even in your forties.

Once you are no longer producing oestrogen, the muscles that support the bladder and control the flow of urine start to weaken. You can no longer hold the urine in quite as effectively as you once did. Hence those awful dribbles.

Whether or not you take HRT (which helps keep the urinary tract in good order), you should be prepared to spend a few minutes a day doing pelvic floor exercises. Remember them? They were the ones you were told to do after you had a baby, but you probably didn't bother. Doing these exercises, also known as Kegel's exercises, helps not only your bladder control, but the whole vaginal area, and so can help your sex life. They are very simple, and you can do them anywhere, at any time. You can do them standing at a bus stop, or at a party, or talking to friends, or watching the television, and no one will ever know you are doing them. Many women start doing them from their thirties onwards, and if they are wise they will certainly be doing them in their forties and fifties. This is what you do:

- Next time you go to the toilet, allow the stream of urine to start, then tighten your muscles to make it stop, and hold the flow for several seconds before releasing it. The muscles you used then are the ones you must now exercise regularly. It is a good routine to do this stopping of the urine several times a day. Perhaps you can only stop the urine for two or three seconds now, but with regular practice you should be able to stop it for ten seconds or even much longer.

Once you know which muscles help to maintain continence, you can exercise them whenever you want. Here are some variations on the same theme:

- Pretend you are stopping the flow of urine, by pulling up these muscles. Hold for a count of five, or 10, or longer if you can, then relax.
- Pull up on the muscles just a little way for a count of three, then pull up further for another count of three, and so on up as many 'steps' as you can. You may manage only one or two 'steps', or you may achieve five or more. Then let the muscles down again, holding each step for a count of three until you have completely relaxed.
- Pull up on the muscles very slowly, and relax very slowly.
- Pull up very quickly, and relax very quickly.

Repeat each exercise about five times in each session, and for several sessions each day. You can probably think of more exercises you can do.

Vaginal dryness

Traditional non-hormonal treatments for vaginal dryness are lubricants such as K-Y Jelly, or a newer product called Replens. These help the symptoms, but do not tackle the underlying cause. Initial penetration will be easier, but prolonged intercourse may be difficult or even impossible as the effect of the lubricant wears off.

Sexual intercourse in the woman-on-top position gives her more control over penetration and how far the penis is inserted, and can make sex more comfortable. It's worth trying different positions, as women who continue to have sex have fewer signs of vaginal ageing than women who don't. Masturbation, too, helps keep the vagina moist and the muscles in good working order. Bear in mind, too, that both men and women take longer to become aroused as they get older. He will take longer to achieve an erection; you will take longer to produce enough mucus. Foreplay may have to go on for longer than it used to, so don't be in a hurry. Take time to reach the state of arousal that will ensure pleasure for both of you.

Sexual feelings, and the production of mucus from the cervix, are greatly affected by how we feel. If you are tense, stressed, depressed or have drunk too much alcohol, don't be surprised if your vagina stays dry. Some medications can alter the sex drive and can affect vaginal dryness – your doctor will be able to advise you about this. Taking more exercise may also help.

Osteoporosis

If you had a premature menopause, especially as the result of the removal of both ovaries, and either can't or won't take HRT, then you should take steps to reduce your chances of getting osteoporosis. The two main medical treatments currently available for osteoporosis that don't involve oestrogen are calcitonin and etidronate.

Calcitonin

This is a naturally occurring hormone that reduces the bone-dissolving activity of the osteoclast cells. It slows the rate of bone loss, and can give a short-term increase in bone density. It is also effective in treating bone pain. However, its effects last for only 18–24 months, so it cannot be taken indefinitely. Also, because it is currently only generally available as an injection, it is very expensive. A nasal spray is undergoing medical trials, and may be available soon; this will still be very expensive, but should be more acceptable.

During childhood, pregnancy and breast-feeding, when bone growth is essential, the body produces extra calcitonin to reduce the action of the osteoclasts, but, like oestrogen, levels drop at the menopause. One way to increase your natural production of this important hormone is to take plenty of exercise in the years around the menopause.

Etidronate

Marketed as Didronel PMO, this is a breakthrough in the non-hormonal treatment of osteoporosis of the spine. It, too, appears to work by reducing the activity of the osteoclasts, and trials show it can lead to a small increase in bone mass and to a reduced risk of fracture. As explained on page 76, it is taken on a cyclical basis: 14 days of etidronate, followed by 76 days of calcium supplements. Etidronate is not the right treatment for everyone, and because it has not been available under general prescription for very long, many GPs are rather uncertain about which patients it is most suitable for, but if you send an s.a.e. to the National Osteoporosis Society (see page 126), they will be able to give you (or your doctor) more information.

Calcium

This mineral has long been recognised as being important for bones, but it is most effective in the years when bones are developing. The post-menopausal woman who swallows great quantities of calcium tablets in the hope of preserving her bones is wasting most of her money. Oestrogen helps to ensure that calcium is absorbed by the body and used effectively, and as oestrogen levels fall much of the calcium is simply excreted in the urine without doing any good. So if you have a daughter in her teens or early twenties, do encourage her to take plenty of calcium in her diet, as this is when it does most good. For yourself, the National Osteoporosis Society recommends the following amounts of calcium a day:

Women over 40, not on HRT	1500 mg
Women over 40 on HRT	1000 mg
Men and women over 60	1200 mg

As a guideline, if you have all of the following each day, you will have had just over 1400 mg of calcium that day, which is ideal:

● a drink of one-third of a pint of semi-skimmed milk,
● one pot of yoghurt,
● milk in a few cups of tea or coffee,
● milk on a bowl of cereal,
● 50 g (2 oz) of Cheddar-type cheese,
● 2 slices of wholemeal bread,
● and a 125 g (4 oz) portion of green leafy vegetables.

If, on the other hand, the only calcium you have is:

● milk in tea or coffee,
● a slice of wholemeal bread,
● 25 g (1 oz) of Cheddar cheese,
● and 125g (4 oz) of green leafy vegetables,

you may think this is a nice low-fat diet and very good for weight control, but it contains only about 440 mg of calcium, so isn't doing your bones any good at all.

After the age of about 35, three-quarters of all women have less than 500 mg of calcium a day, many of these being post-menopausal women not on HRT who should be having three times that amount. Unfortunately, as they get older, women tend to take less and less calcium, just when they should be taking more. So if you are worried about 'middle-aged spread', don't cut down on dairy products, try instead to use skimmed or semi-skimmed milk (which are higher in calcium and lower in fat than ordinary milk), to eat more fruit, vegetables and starch, less fat, and less alcohol.

Exercise

It is also important to take plenty of exercise to burn off the excess calories and to strengthen your bones. The more bones and muscles are used, the stronger they grow, so from your middle years onwards the new buzz-words in your life should be 'mechanical loading', which means giving your bones plenty of work. As you use your muscles, the bone-building osteoblasts respond by building more bone; exercise is also thought to stimulate the production of calcitonin, thereby slowing the activity of the bone-dissolving osteoclasts. We have only as much bone as we need, and nothing will cause the skeleton to become stronger than it needs to be for your lifestyle. No amount of calcium tablets will compensate for 'mechanical loading' of the bones and muscles.

Exercise is something most of us do much less of as we get older, which is a pity, as it:

• helps to build up bones
• is good for the heart
• reduces depression and stress
• improves muscle tone and co-ordination, so reducing the risk of falling (which is one of the main causes of fractures)
• is an effective form of weight control
• improves sleep

All these things become more important after the menopause, so try to build some regular exercise into your life. If you have already had an osteoporotic fracture, you should take advice from your specialist or from a physiotherapist about what form of exercise you should and should not be taking. If you have no sign of this disease, then you should be having plenty of exercise that loads the bones and muscles. Swimming and yoga are very good for all the other aspects of your life, but as they do not put any strain on bones you would need to include some other forms of exercise as well, such as tennis, dancing, brisk walking, aerobics, fitness training, etc.

Just a word of caution: forget the old maxim 'If it isn't hurting, it isn't working'; after about the age of 35 this is a harmful philosophy, so listen to your body, and when it says 'stop', then stop before you do some damage you will regret.

The role of supplements

Like facial moisturisers, dietary supplements are a multi-pound industry. Your local health food shop will stock pills and potions for every conceivable condition, including numerous products especially packaged for women – vitamins and minerals, Royal Jelly, ginseng, evening primrose oil. Most of the 'alternative' remedies have not been subjected to the rigorous testing that conventional medicines have to undergo, and some of them may cause side-effects such as headaches and stomach upsets. Many women do find them helpful, however, especially for menstrual problems, sleeplessness and lethargy, so they should not be dismissed. Many of them work on the placebo effect, that is they work because you want them to work, and if taking a dietary supplement makes your hot flushes less troublesome, then that is what is important.

If you are thinking of trying alternative remedies for menopausal problems, a qualified alternative practitioner might be the best person to visit. On page 125 you will find a list of addresses through which you can find homoeopaths, acupuncturists, medical herbalists, osteopaths and hypnotherapists with well recognised and respected qualifications.

Most of the menopausal symptoms discussed in this book are caused by one main thing – a fall in the level of oestrogen – and herbal remedies cannot replace oestrogen. You may have seen advertisements in newspapers and magazines for substances which call themselves 'Herbal Hormone Replacement Therapy', which claim to replace male and female hormones, and to provide equivalent benefits to HRT as prescribed by doctors. They don't! Following some test-case complaints, in 1991 the Advertising Standards Authority (ASA) ruled that the manufacturers concerned had failed to submit any documentation that proved the products could provide any benefit to the customer, and the ASA was particularly concerned that the advertisements might lead people to buy the product instead of visiting a doctor. In the cases concerned, the manufacturers were requested to withdraw the advertisements and not to make any further claims for their products until they were able to substantiate them completely.

So go cautiously when considering over-the-counter remedies for menopausal symptoms. Some work, some don't. Take care to take only the recommended dose: if it says 'one tablet a day', then don't think the remedy will be twice as effective if you take two tablets a day; it won't, and that dose may be harmful. It is easier to take too much of a nutrient in tablet form than it is from foods, and too much of one nutrient can cause an imbalance in others, which may make your symptoms worse. Try not to become dependent on them, or to make them a substitute for a good diet and lifestyle.

Chapter 10

How you see yourself

Women in parts of India who are kept in purdah welcome the arrival of the menopause as an era of new freedom; now they can cast off their veils, mix with men and travel freely. In China, the sixtieth birthday is a momentous event, celebrating the status and wisdom of the old person. After the menopause, Bantu women may take part in activities previously forbidden to them, and women in Bali can join in ceremonies from which they were barred during their childbearing years. From India to Africa, from China to South America, the end of menstruation brings new freedom to women. Middle-aged and elderly women are an active part of the extended family, they help on the land, they feel useful, needed and valued. Ageing is a gain in wisdom, not just the loss of youth; in the same way that many cultures celebrate the start of a girl's menstruation, so its ending is a positive event, too. And in countries where older people have enhanced privilege and status, menopausal symptoms are almost unknown.

How different things are in our 'advanced' societies of the West. Ours is a society that gives status and emphasis to physical prowess, to attractiveness and to youth. Men and women (but especially men) lose status when they are no longer defined by the job they do. Children grow up and move away, and the busy mother/chauffeur/cook/nanny/ supporter of the PTA/and helper at Brownies suddenly finds her role has disappeared. In these societies, where getting older is seen as a definite minus, 80 per cent of women suffer from menopausal symptoms.

You probably remember the days when 'black' was a term of abuse towards people of African and Caribbean origin. Most black people living in white cultures at that time felt themselves to be inferior to whites, accepting their status as second-class citizens. Then black people themselves coined the phrase 'Black is Beautiful', and suddenly their image changed. They felt proud of their black heritage and culture, and of the colour of their skin.

Why shouldn't older people, too, change how they see themselves, and how society sees them? The Gray Panther movement in the United States is a powerful lobby for the rights of retired people, and they certainly don't see themselves as has-beens.

There are now 10 million women over the age of 50 in the UK – that's 17 per cent of the population . . . and rising. By the year 2000, that 10 million will have become 14 million. Middle-aged women nowadays are a group with changed expectations. The menopause may have been hidden for our mothers and grandmothers, but not for us. We are no longer willing to be silent on important aspects of our lives, whether it is employment opportunities, taxation, child care, equal rights and responsibilities, or anything medical. We expect our doctors to be well-informed, and to share that information with us as equals. We may still get the flushes, the sweats, and perhaps eventually the osteoporosis, but now we know what causes them, and that they can be prevented – or at least reduced. It needn't be the same for us as it was for our mothers.

This is now a good time for women of 50-ish and more to assert themselves, to make themselves visible. A woman reaching her fiftieth birthday in the mid-1990s is part of the post-war baby boom, who, to the envy of her children, was right there in the Swinging Sixties. She is part of such a large population bulge that she is being noticed. Advertisers reach out to her, car insurance companies devise special policies for her, she can buy magazines aimed at her age group, and she can join clubs that bear no resemblance to the local Darby and Joan. If it was good to be a young woman in the Sixties, it's just as good to be a middle-aged woman now. There have never been more examples of women in their forties, fifties, and beyond, who are attractive and confident, pursuing exciting, demanding careers, often earning more than their husbands do, real Women at the Top.

Other people's attitudes towards you may change as you get older, but they will only belittle you if you let them. You will only be ignored if you let yourself be.

❛I went into a restaurant with my elderly mother, and we started to sit down at one of the many empty tables in the front of the restaurant. A waiter appeared and showed us to a table at the back of the restaurant right near the kitchen door. When I asked if we could have one of the front tables, he said they were all reserved. He took our coats, brought two menus and left us to choose our meal. But we weren't happy in that dark out-of-the-way position, and when he came back to take our order, I said that we did not like this table, and please would he bring our coats as we were leaving. Well, lo and behold!, suddenly those tables were not all reserved after all, and he invited us to choose which one of them we would like to sit at. I have since discovered that women on their own are often given second-rate tables in restaurants, but I'll never let that happen to me again!❜

By being assertive and standing up for yourself, you help not only yourself, but all other older women, too. Until a few years ago, most women would choose not to tell anyone they had reached their fortieth birthday; now you see banners across the streets of towns and villages proclaiming messages such as 'Happy 40th Birthday, Susan', and suddenly Susan is happy to admit she is 40, and is not ashamed of it.

You, too, can be proud of your age; once everyone around you is also admitting they are 50-something, then that will be seen to be a good age, as will 60-something and 70-something. Feeling ashamed of your age can lead to a low self-esteem, and this is a time of life to do all you can to bolster your self-esteem. Middle-aged women are just as interesting as younger women, and not a jot less interesting than middle-aged men. If you believe you are interesting, other people will share that belief; if you think you are a dull boring old person, you will convey that feeling to everyone you meet. If other cultures can find older women wise and interesting and important in society, our culture can, too, and it is up to us to set the ball rolling.

Women who find older people boring and invisible will dread their own advancing age, and will manage it badly. So feel attractive, believe in yourself and what you can do, and you won't notice the passing of the years so much. Today is the first day of the rest of your life, and it's not too late to start anything. If you wanted to, you could take up hang-gliding, learn Portuguese, start your own business, teach pottery, travel anywhere in the world. If you feel trapped in an unhappy marriage, you could even leave your husband if you felt that was the right thing to do, and you can certainly remake your own life if he leaves you. The more you feel you are in control of your own life, the happier you will be.

Talk to other women of your age about how you are feeling. Share your worries, your embarrassment about hot flushes, even your anxieties and feelings about how your sex life may be changing. Knowing other women are feeling as you do will make you feel less isolated and much better in yourself.

When I am an old woman I shall wear purple
With a red hat which doesn't go, and doesn't suit me.
And I shall spend my pension on brandy and summer gloves
And satin sandals, and say we've no money for butter.
I shall sit down on the pavement when I am tired
And gobble up samples in shops and press alarm bells
And run my stick along the public railings
And make up for the sobriety of my youth.
I shall go out in my slippers in the rain

And pick the flowers in other people's gardens
And learn to spit.

You can wear terrible shirts and grow more fat
And eat three pounds of sausages at a go
Or only bread and pickle for a week
And hoard pens and pencils and beermats and things in boxes.

But now we must have clothes that keep us dry
And pay the rent and not swear in the street
And set a good example for the children.
We must have friends to dinner and read the papers.

But maybe I ought to practise a little now?
So people who know me are not too shocked and surprised
When suddenly I am old and start to wear purple.

Rose in The Afternoon by Jenny Joseph
(from *Selected Poems*, Bloodaxe Books Ltd. © Jenny Joseph 1992)

* * *

Whether you decide to take hormone replacement therapy
is a decision you will need to make after talking to your
doctor, to your friends who may have tried it, and after
weighing the pros and cons. There is little doubt that, taking the population as a whole, the benefits far outweigh the
risks, but for you as an individual the balance may be different. It will depend, for example, on how you feel about
the risks of breast cancer versus the risks of osteoporosis or
heart disease, on how severe your menopausal symptoms
are versus the side-effects you get on HRT, and on how
you feel about taking hormones. How do you balance an
immediate improvement in your quality of life against the
long-term risks, especially of breast cancer? How much
would you risk the possibility of side-effects now and breast
cancer later to gain the many other benefits it brings? As a
general rule, we tend to be more worried about taking a
treatment that has an increased risk of disease than about
failing to take a treatment that could decrease the risks of
other conditions.

Oestrogen replacement therapy has been available since the 1940s, and its beneficial effects have been well documented since the 1950s. Yet, over 40 years later, fear and confusion among both doctors and their patients is still preventing the majority of women from receiving – or continuing with – a treatment that can enormously improve so many aspects of their lives.

The eminent British gynaecologist, John Studd, has described oestrogen therapy for post-menopausal women as:

‘probably the most important advance in preventive medicine in the Western world for half a century, with fewer heart attacks, fewer strokes, fewer osteoporotic fractures, less depression and an extra year or two of life.’

This is how some women sum up their own personal experiences of HRT:

‘I know many people feel women should be able to struggle on without it, or use more natural remedies. All I know is that it has made all the difference to how I feel, and to my life in general.’

‘After taking HRT for a few months I decided to stop, because I felt it was unnatural and I didn’t think I really needed it. All my symptoms came back and I started to feel quite unwell again, so I went back on it. I feel great now, but I’m not completely happy that I only feel really well if I keep taking the hormones.’

‘I was developing a lot of unexpected aches and pains, and intercourse was uncomfortable and ‘dry’, and I wasn’t really interested in it. My joints feel much more supple since I started taking HRT; and intercourse has become a pleasure again.’

‘I was given an implant after a hysterectomy at the age of 45. Before then I had been suffering from aching joints and tiredness. Now I feel fine. I know that a few women with implants can become ‘dependent’ on it because it makes them feel so good, but that hasn’t happened to me.’

‘Taking HRT was my doctor’s idea, and I feel I’m lucky to have a doctor who believes in it and who has been prepared to keep trying to find the one that suits me best.’

'I hope it will give me a good quality of life.'

'I am my old self again.'

'There is a new vitality about me that I thought had gone forever. I had some side-effects at first, but they soon wore off, and my doctor has been tremendously helpful and supportive all the time.'

'How does it make me feel? In a word – brilliant.'

Glossary of medical terms

abdomen the belly; that part of the body between the bottom of the ribs and the groin area

adrenal glands a pair of glands, each situated on top of a kidney

amenorrhoea absence of periods

androgens hormones that produce male characteristics in either sex

anorexia nervosa a condition in which the sufferer diets drastically to lose real or imagined weight; 'the slimmers' disease'

arterial disease disease of the arteries, notably heart attack and stroke

atrophy wasting away through lack of use or nutrition

benign not cancerous

bone density a measure of the amount of mineral (mainly calcium) in a bone

bone loss the process of losing bone density

bone mass the total quantity of calcium-rich bone

bulimia a condition in which the sufferer binges on large quantities of food, and then vomits, as a means of losing real or imaginary weight

cardio-vascular concerning the heart and circulatory system

cholesterol a blood fat

climacteric the years around the menopause, before and after the final period, when menopausal symptoms are being experienced

collagen part of the skin; part of the bone in which calcium is deposited

continence control of the bladder and bowel

continuous-combined HRT a form of HRT in which oestrogens and progestogens are both taken continuously

contraindication a reason for considering that a particular treatment is unsuitable, usually because it will make an existing condition worse

cortical bone the hard outer layer of all bones

cystitis inflammation of the lining of the bladder

dyspareunia painful sexual intercourse

endometrial cancer cancer of the endometrium

endometrial hyperplasia non-cancerous overgrowth of tissue in the endometrium

endometrium the lining of the uterus

ERT estrogen replacement therapy (US)

estrogen American spelling of oestrogen

fibroids non-cancerous tumours in the wall of the uterus

formication a feeling of insects crawling under or on top of the skin

frequency needing to pass urine frequently

gastro-intestinal concerning the digestive organs

genito-urinary atrophy atrophy of the genital and urinary tract

gynaecologist a doctor who specialises in the treatment and management of disorders affecting the female organs

high density lipoproteins (HDLs) a form of cholesterol that, among other things, attaches to low density lipoproteins (LDLs) and allows them to be absorbed out of blood vessels

hormone a chemical substance that is produced in one part of the body and acts on other parts

hot flash American term for 'hot flush'

hot flush sudden flow of heat to the skin

hysterectomy surgical removal of the uterus, sometimes also including the cervix and ovaries

implant a form of HRT in which a small pellet containing hormones is inserted under the skin

incontinence loss of control of the bladder or bowel

Kegel exercises pelvic floor exercises to aid continence

libido sex drive, interest in sex

low density lipoproteins (LDLs) a form of cholesterol that can become attached to the walls of blood vessels, thereby restricting the flow of blood

menopausal relating to the menopause

menopause medically speaking, the final period; most women use it to define that part of their lives when they experience menopausal symptoms

menstrual cycle the time from the start of one menstrual period to the beginning of the next

menstruation the monthly bleed (period) that occurs in non-pregnant females between puberty and the menopause

natural menopause a menopause that occurs naturally, without surgery or drugs

nausea feeling sick

no-bleed HRT a form of HRT in which a 'withdrawal bleed' does not occur

nocturia needing to pass urine during the night

non-oral route a way of taking treatment that does not involve the mouth; with HRT this means patches, implants, gels and creams instead of tablets

obesity excessive overweight

oestrogen the hormone responsible for female sexual characteristics, produced by the ovaries; forms of oestrogen are beta-oestradiol, oestrone and oestriol

oestrogen deficiency being low in oestrogen

oestrogen receptors areas of an organ that respond to the presence of oestrogen

oestrone, oestradiol, oestriol forms of the female hormone oestrogen

oophorectomy removal of one ovary (unilateral oophorectomy) or both ovaries (bilateral oophorectomy)

oral HRT a form of HRT that is taken by mouth (tablets)

osteoblasts cells within the bone that form new bone by a constant process of rebuilding and repairing

osteoclasts cells within the bone that dissolve old bone so that it can be replaced by the osteoblasts

osteoporosis a disease in which bone becomes so porous, brittle and fragile that it breaks very easily

ovaries two small organs on either side of the abdomen in which the female sex hormones oestrogen and progesterone are produced, and from which an ovum (egg) is produced each month during the reproductive years

ovulation the production of an ovum (egg) from the ovaries

patch a form of HRT in which hormones are absorbed through the skin from a stick-on patch

peak bone mass the maximum amount of calcium-rich bone an individual achieves, usually by the age of 30–35

peri-menopause the time in a woman's life when she starts to experience menopausal symptoms but still has periods, although they become steadily more irregular

post-menopause after the final period

premature menopause a menopause that occurs before about the age of 45, whether natural or surgical

pre-menopause before menopausal systems and irregular periods start

pre-menstrual syndrome (PMS) physical and psychological symptoms that many women experience in the days leading up to menstruation

progesterone a naturally occurring female hormone

progestogen a synthetic form of progesterone

puberty the period of sexual development

risk the likelihood that a condition will develop as a direct result of medical treatment

route in the case of HRT this means the method by which it is taken, ie oral, transdermal, subcutaneous

site in the case of HRT this means the area of the body from which the hormones are absorbed (abdomen, thigh, buttocks)

stress incontinence leakage of urine when sneezing, coughing, laughing or taking vigorous exercise

subcutaneous HRT HRT that is absorbed from under the skin, an implant

surgical menopause a menopause that occurs as a result of surgery, rather than naturally; a hysterectomy or oophorectomy

symptom a noticeable change in the body and the way it works, usually as felt by the patient

tachyphylaxis in the case of HRT, this is a condition in which some women with implants experience a return of menopausal symptoms even though their blood oestrogen levels are normal or high

testosterone the male sexual hormone, secreted by the testes

trabecular bone the inner layer of bones that is at risk in osteoporosis

tranquilliser a drug that has a calming sedative effect

transdermal HRT a form of HRT in which the hormones are absorbed through the skin; the patch

urethra the tube that carries urine from the bladder to outside the body

urgency needing to pass water urgently

uterus the womb

vagina the birth canal; the passage leading from the base of the uterus to outside the body

vaginitis infection or inflammation of the vagina

vasomotor symptoms symptoms caused by constriction of blood vessels; in the case of HRT this refers to hot flushes, night sweats, and also to some forms of headache

vertebra, vertebrae (plural) the bones which form the backbone, or spine

withdrawal bleed loss of blood from the uterus caused when a course of progestogen is completed

Useful addresses

Charities and voluntary organisations always appreciate the enclosure of a stamped addressed envelope when you write to them.

Action on Smoking and Health (ASH), 5–11 Mortimer Street, London W1N 7RH (Tel: 071–637 9843)

Age Concern, Astral House, 1268 London Road, London SW16 4EJ (Tel: 081–679 8000)

Amarant Trust (information and advice on the menopause and HRT), Grant House, 56–60 St John Street, London EC1M 4DT (Tel: 071–490 1644). HRT Helpline Tel: 0338–400190

Association of Continence Advisors, 380–384 Harrow Road, London W9 2HU (Tel: 071–289 6111)

Breast Care and Mastectomy Association of Great Britain, 26a Harrison Street, Kings Cross, London WC1H 8JG (Tel: 071–867 1103)

British Heart Foundation, 102 Gloucester Place, London W1H 4DH (Tel: 071–935 0185)

British Homoeopathic Association, 27a Devonshire Street, London W1N 1JR (Tel: 071–935 2163) – for list of medically qualified homoeopaths

Continence Helpline – 091–213 0050

The Council for Acupuncture, 179 Gloucester Place, London NW1 6DX (Tel: 071–724 5756)

Cruse (bereavement care), Cruse House, 126 Sheen Road, Richmond, Surrey TW9 1UR (Tel: 081–940 4818)

Family Planning Association, 27–35 Mortimer Street, London W1N 7RJ (Tel: 071–636 7866)

General Council and Register of Osteopaths, 56 London Street, Reading, Berks RG1 4SQ (Tel: 0734–576585)

Hysterectomy Support Group, 11 Henryson Road, London SE4 (Tel: 081–690 5987)

Institute for Complementary Medicine, 21 Portland Place, London W1 (Tel: 071–636 9543)

Institute of Psychosexual Medicine, 11 Chandos Street, Cavendish Square, London W1M 9DE (Tel: 071–580 0631)

National Association of Widows, 54–57 Alison Street, Digbeth, Birmingham B5 5TH (Tel: 021–643 8343)

National Back Pain Association, 31–33 Park Road, Teddington, Middx TW11 0AB (Tel: 081–977 5474)

National Institute of Medical Herbalists, 9 Palace Gate, Exeter, Devon EX1 1JA (Tel: 0392–426022)

National Osteoporosis Society, PO Box 10, Radstock, Bath BA3 3YB (Tel: 0671–432472). Helpline Tel: 0761–431594

Relate (National Marriage Guidance Council), Herbert Gray College, Little Church Street, Rugby, Warwickshire CV21 3AP (Tel: 0788–573241)

Relaxation for Living, 29 Burwood Park Road, Walton on Thames, Surrey KY12 5LH

The Society of Homoeopaths, 2 Artisan Road, Northampton NN1 4HU (Tel: 0604–21400) – for lay homoeopaths, not medically qualified

Women's Health Concern, PO Box 1629, London W8 6AU (Tel: 071–938 3932)

Women's National Cancer Control Campaign, 1 South Audley Street, London W1 (Tel: 071–499 7532)

Index

facial hair, 5, 45
fats:
  cholesterol, 27–8, 37
  oestrogen production by fat
    cells, 4–5
  progestrogen and, 37
fibroids, 89, 120
fluid retention, 82
flushes *see* hot flushes
formication, 23, 120
fractures, 67–8, 70, 72–3
frequency, 120

gallbladder, 87
gallstones, 89
gastro-intestinal disturbances, 83,
  120
gels, 40, 49–50
genito-urinary atrophy, 120
Gray Panthers, 112
gum problems, 26
gynaecological check-ups, 85–6
gynaecologists, 120

hair:
  facial, 5, 45
  hair loss, 23, 26
headaches, 84, 90
heart attacks, 27, 37, 62, 87, 96–7
heart disease, 88
herbal remedies, 101, 109–10
high blood pressure, 89
high density lipoproteins (HDL),
  27–8, 120
hips:
  bone density, 69
  fractures, 68, 70, 72–3
homoeopaths, 101
hormone replacement therapy
  (HRT):
  and breast cancer, 94–8
  continuous/combined, 36, 50
  contraindications, 86–90
  creams and gels, 47–50

disadvantages of, 79–86
disadvantages of progestogen,
  31–8
doctors and, 90–3
dosages, 51–2
and hot flushes, 16–17
how to stop taking, 55–6
how to take, 39–52
implants, 44–7
'no-bleed' HRT, 36–7, 50, 85
and osteoporosis, 72–3, 76–8
patches, 42–4
risk factors, 115
and sexuality, 58–9, 64
side-effects, 51–2, 81–4
symptoms after stopping, 56–7
tablets, 41–2
when to start taking, 52–5
see also oestrogen; progestogen
hormones, 120
  androgens, 4–5, 50, 119
  calcitonin, 105–6, 108
  functions, 2–4
  progesterone, 4, 32
  testosterone, 3, 4, 45, 64–5
  see also oestrogen; progestogen
hot flushes, 120
  causes, 13–18
  duration of, 54
  HRT and, 16–18, 52, 84
  stopping HRT, 42, 56–7
  treatment without HRT, 100–1
hysterectomy, 31, 84, 120
  hormonal effects, 9–10
  HRT dosages, 51, 53
  implants and, 47
  oophorectomy, 10, 51, 53, 69,
    88–9
  ovaries after, 9–10

implants, 40, 44–7, 56, 64, 121
impotence, 65
incontinence, 23, 25, 54–5, 103–4,
  121

If you have enjoyed this book, you may also be interested in the following titles published by Vermilion:

Beat PMT Through Diet   : £6.99
Beat PMT Cookbook   : £6.99
Beat Sugar Craving   : £6.99
Getting Sober and Loving It   : £6.99
How to Stop Smoking   : £5.99
The Complete Guide to Psychiatric Drugs   : £7.99
Lyn Marshall's Instant Stress Cure   : £7.99

To obtain your copy, simply telephone Murlyn Services on

0279 427203

You may pay by cheque/postal order/VISA and should allow 28 days for delivery. Postage and packing is free.